Psychosocial Interventions for Chronic Pain

Ranjan Roy

Psychosocial Interventions for Chronic Pain

In Search of Evidence

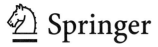 Springer

Ranjan Roy
University of Manitoba
Winnipeg, Canada
rroy@cc.umanitoba.ca

ISBN: 978-0-387-76295-1   e-ISBN: 978-0-387-76296-8
DOI: 10.1007/978-0-387-76296-8

Library of Congress Control Number: 2008921455

Printed on acid-free paper

9 8 7 6 5 4 3 2 1

springer.com

For my friend Dr. Brian Minty of the University of Manchester for his friendship and support in all my academic endeavours

Preface

The idea for this monograph came to me following a review of my book *Chronic Pain, Loss and Grief* by Professor Harold Merskey, a leading figure in the field of chronic pain. He wrote that he was happy to see a book that had departed from the idea of "one treatment (Cognitive Behavioral Therapy: CBT) fits all." This volume is an exploration of psychosocial interventions beyond, but not excluding, CBT that may be used to one degree or another by the practitioners in the field. And the related question is, "How good are they?" Another fact that contributed to the actual shape of this book emerged from my graduate seminars on psychotherapy with individuals. One aspect of that course is to consider the evidence for each and every kind of psychotherapy that students choose to discuss. Contribution of my students in the development and shaping of this volume is beyond measure, and I take this opportunity to thank them.

It has to be acknowledged at the outset that the dominance of CBT in treating chronic pain patients and the evidence to justify its application is impressive. Numerous randomized controlled trials (RCTs) testify to that (see Chapter 8). Yet, CBT is not a panacea. Our research also revealed that many practitioners, including myself, were engaged in implementing a wide variety of psychotherapeutic interventions with or without the benefit of strong empirical evidence. At times such evidence was close to nonexistent, particularly when judged against RCTs, the gold standard for all outcomes. However, other kinds of evidence such as clinical or qualitative or less sophisticated quantitative methodology were offered to justify the choice of therapy. We have included such interventions. One critical question that all psychotherapists must ask is the fit between a particular problem and the choice of therapy. A common problem that confronts all therapists is not always having the information about the rationale behind the choice of therapy. Are there clear or as clear as possible guidelines about patient characteristics or the problems that may determine the choice of therapy? More often than not, there is no such guideline. Is it possible that the dominance of CBT to treat chronic pain has had a dampening effect on research to explore the effectiveness of other types of psychotherapeutic interventions? Our research suggests that indeed that may be the case. So, we cast a wide net and report on many and varied psychotherapeutic interventions that have been used to one extent or another to treat chronic pain sufferers. It is our hope that clinicians will give consideration to the choices available to them.

As for research evidence, a number of therapies discussed in this volume are wanting, and because the evidence is poor or inadequate, there is little or no impetus for research. This cycle needs to break. Another related issue is that different therapeutic interventions claim (justifiably) to be effective in treating a particular problem. An example of that would be the effectiveness of CBT, interpersonal psychotherapy (IPT), or psychodynamically oriented psychotherapy in treating grief related to loss. Unless convincing evidence emerges to show the superiority, or otherwise, of one over the other, the selection of one therapy over another becomes a matter of personal choice. Only research can settle the matter.

This book has 11 chapters. Chapter 1 addresses in broad terms the pros and cons of an evidence-based psychosocial approach. It would appear that although the value of evidence-based approach is widely acknowledged, its application is less than universal. Research-based practice for psychotherapists engaged in treating chronic pain sufferers or medically ill patients may not be the rule. Evidence of the effectiveness of many psychotherapeutic interventions is not always convincing. This could be a function of the very high scientific requirement of what might be considered acceptable evidence, should other kinds of evidence, such as qualitative or even quantitative (falling below the rigor of CBT), be taken into account. We discuss the effectiveness of solution-focused therapy (SFT), a widely used method by clinical social workers, to deal with a multitude of psychosocial problems.

Chapter 2 is a consideration of the nature and extent of psychosocial problems commonly encountered by our patients. A critical question that emerges from this pursuit is the choice of therapy we often make to treat our patients. More broadly, do the therapies we use succeed in alleviating or even eliminating the psychosocial problems?

Chapters 3 through 10 present different types of psychotherapeutic interventions that may be used to one degree or another to treat our patients. We preface these chapters, where possible, with case illustrations. An intervention such as CBT is widely used and derives its strength from solid research. Other interventions, such as family therapy or psychodynamic psychotherapy, are reported in the literature, but the evidence for their effectiveness is somewhat wanting. Nevertheless, our objective is simply to offer a rationale for their application and urge for more research.

Chapter 11 tries to focus on the state of the art, highlighting the trends and the gaps. We also urge an open-mindedness in the choice of therapy, and a shift in focus to further refine the notion of matching therapy with the problems. Even CBT, for all its success, is not a panacea.

This project may not have materialized without the encouragement and support of my wife, Margaret. As always, she helped me in numerous tangible and intangible ways to finish this book. She has my undying gratitude and love. I also want to thank Dr. Michael Thomas, my friend and research partner for over 25 years. Without his friendship and patience, much of our work could not have been accomplished. Thank you, Michael!

About the Author

Ranjan Roy is Professor in the Faculty of Social Work and Department of Clinical Health Psychology, University of Manitoba, Winnipeg, Canada. He is also a consultant (scientific) in the Department of Anesthesiology, Health Sciences Center, Winnipeg. Ranjan Roy is Fellow of the Royal Society of Canada, Canadian Academy of Arts, Science, and Social Science. He has published extensively on the psychosocial aspects of chronic pain.

Contents

Chapter 1
Evidence-Based Approach and Psychosocial Practice

Evidence-based approach to psychosocial problems has come under sustained exploration in the last decade or so. Although psychosocial issues do not have the refinement of medical diagnosis and treatment, they are nevertheless not unamenable to such scrutiny and desirable standard. First, we shall examine the applicability of evidence-based approach to the treatment of psychosocial problems. Second, we examine the problems associated with the classification (taxonomy) of psychosocial problems. Finally, we consider the question of appropriate therapies for treating the psychosocial problems.

Evidence-Based Practice and Its Relevance to Psychosocial Problems

In the past two decades or so evidence-based practice (EBP) in medicine has achieved a central place. In the medical literature, not too much criticism is found on EBP. Since Sackett's seminal work in which he laid out the principles of EBP in the practice of medicine, it has gathered momentum in many health-related professions.

Sackett et al. (1977, p. 2) defined EBP as "the conscientious, explicit, and judicious use of the current best evidence in making decisions about the care of individual patients." This definition leaves considerable latitude in the quality of evidence and, in fact, creates a hierarchy of evidence. Nevertheless, another cogent definition was provided by the American Surgeon General Dr. David Schacter who proclaimed that "All things considered, evidence-based treatment is treatment based upon the best available science" (NPR broadcast, December 13, 1999). Although randomized controlled trials (RCTs) may be regarded as the gold standard of practice, in the psychotherapeutic arena their requirements would be hard to fulfill should clinical evidence, which may be based on a collection of reports, on a particular treatment, and beyond that qualitative data be considered "the available science."

R. Roy, *Psychosocial Interventions for Chronic Pain*,
DOI: 10.1007/978-0-387-76296-8_1 © Springer Science+Business Media, LLC 2008

Thyer and Kazi (2004) presented the following guidelines for evidence-based practitioners:

- Provide informed consent for treatment
- Rely on efficacy data (especially from RCTs) when recommending and selecting and carrying out treatment
- Use the empirical literature to guide decision making
- Use a systematic hypothesis-testing approach to the treatment of each case

  - Begin with a careful assessment
  - Set clear and measurable goals
  - Develop an individualized formulation and a treatment plan based on that formulation
  - Monitor progress toward the goals frequently
  - Modify and end treatment as needed

There are several assumptions underlying these guidelines that will presently come under some scrutiny.

Medicine has a long tradition of science-driven practice. Establishment of diagnostic taxonomy has a time-honored tradition of rigorous scientific investigation and there always is a direct link between diagnosis and treatment. In the psychosocial arena neither the diagnosis nor the treatment has any such link. Yet, the 1995 American Psychological Association (APA) Division 12 Task Force on the Promotion and Dissemination of Psychological Procedures (Chambless, 1995; Chambless et al., 1998) established that as a precondition for treatment, its efficacy must include the following:

- At least two good between-group design experiments demonstrating efficacy in at least one of the following ways:

  - superior to pill or psychological placebo or to another treatment in experiments with adequate sample sizes and/or
  - equivalent to an already established treatment in experiments with adequate sample sizes.

- A large series of single-case designs demonstrating efficacy in the following ways:

  - used good experimental designs and
  - compared the intervention with another treatment.

Generally speaking, clinical psychologists rely on the Diagnostic and Statistical Manual of Mental Disorders, Fourth Edition (DSM-IV) for diagnosing their patients. As we purport to show in the following section, not all psychosocial problems are amenable to such diagnosis and therefore, interventions lack the level of clarity demanded by strict adherence to the criteria discussed above.

Despite some obvious problems in the implementation of EBP, there is an emerging body of literature in social work that strongly advocates its adoption in social work practice. This is an encouraging development as social work, of all healthcare professions, is almost exclusively focused on psychosocial or, more precisely, on social problems. We provide a brief summary of that literature below.

There exists a great deal of philosophical debate within the social work community about the desirability of EBP (Sheldon, 2001; Smith, 2004; Webb, 2001). Here we avoid that debate to examine the quality of data that may support incorporation of EBP in social work practice. In this context, we examine two major publications that explore the application of EBP: one from an international perspective (Thyer and Kazi, 2004) and the other on its application to various practice settings (Smith, 2004).

Thyer and Kazi (2004) produced a collection of essays that reported on varying levels of success with EBP from the United Kingdom (England, Scotland, and Northern Ireland) and six other countries (United States, Canada, Australia, China, South Africa, and Finland). It is not easy to assess the level of implementation of EBP in all these countries with a very wide range of social problems. However, it can be stated with some certainty that EBP is far from universal in social work practice. There is also wide variability between the countries. Canada, for example, lags considerably behind the United States both in EBP-based social work education and in practice. In fact, many social work academics remain suspect of the value of EBP, and regard it as a governmental instrument to control social spending.

We chose the two countries reported in Thyer and Kazi's book to compare the development of EBP to address social problems: the United States, the largest country (in the book), and Finland, one of the smallest countries. We confine our observations to EBP in practice settings, which provide us with a realistic picture of the range of problems for which EBP have met with favorable outcome.

Thyer (2004) in his assessment of the state of EBP in the United States noted that actual EBP is far from widespread. In fact, close scrutiny of his chapter leaves a clear impression that application of EBP in treating major social problems by social workers, in the main, remains elusive. In fact, Thyer (2004), rather ruefully noted that "Unfortunately for social workers and other non-physician providers of healthcare, the APA practice guidelines tend to overemphasize pharmacotherapy at the expense of psychosocial treatment" (p. 34).

One major development has been the establishment of the Campbell Collaboration, with the goal of conducting systematic reviews of research in the social welfare, criminal justice, and educational problems. However, Thyer noted that at the time of writing (2004) Campbell Collaboration had not undertaken a single review. Thyer's (2004) final observations are poignant indeed: "... it must be acknowledged that most contemporary professional social workers in the USA are not very familiar with the concepts of EBP, and fewer still provide care guided by these principles" (pp. 36–37).

Thyer observed that the profession of social work tends to be involved in extraordinarily complex social structures such as the poor, the minorities of color, and other historically oppressed groups, which make the application of RCTs a very challenging activity. It is noteworthy that the types of problems Thyer identified as being in the domain of social work are also firmly rooted in the political and economic arenas. The point is that no individual intervention is capable of eradicating any of these problems. On the contrary, when individuals are faced with specific issues of discrimination or poverty due to a change in their particular circumstances, specifically defined interventions are possible. Our endeavor throughout this volume will be to examine these individual-based interventions.

The situation in Finland, if anything, is even less promising than in the United States. Social work research in critical fields such as rehabilitation was mainly absent (Rostila and Piirainen, 2004). The authors lamented the fact that research related to client systems and their environment was sparse. However, research on the effectiveness of rehabilitation of the long-term unemployed and seniors in the Finnish society has been extensive, although the research was not necessarily conducted by social workers. Similarly, the outcome of treatment for alcoholics in terms of their social inclusion and reemployment is promising. The authors also noted that "Knowledge-building about outcomes and effectiveness in social work, including research done by social workers or social work researchers ... is largely absent" (p. 201).

Throughout Thyer and Kazi's book there is a twofold acknowledgment: (1) absence of research to promote EBP for social workers and (2) the necessity of doing so. Multitude of explanations are offered for this state of affairs, but the future of EBP in social work is seen as promising. One aspect that remained unaddressed in this book was the need to develop a classification system for social problems from which will flow a critical examination of effective interventions. Even a cursory examination of the literature would reveal a persistent effort to develop such a taxonomy. The proposition is simple. It is virtually impossible to develop appropriate interventions in the absence of well-defined problems. In medicine, treatment follows from diagnosis. In the social arena, perhaps the social problems can never have the precision of a medical diagnosis, but some broad classification of these problems will lead to the development of specific treatments. In the following section, we review the most recent literature on the efforts that have gone into the development of a taxonomy for social problems.

Taxonomy for Social Problems: A Selected Literature Review

What may constitute a psychosocial problem? Oxford English Dictionary defines "psychosocial" as involving the influence of social factors on human interactive behavior. The term is used to convey any and all kinds of problems that fall outside the domain of medicine. The underlying assumption, however, is that social and psychological problems exist in a manner that makes separating them a hazardous task. On the one hand, social problems are experienced at a personal level, be it unemployment or truancy or a sudden loss, which almost always have psychological concomitants, and may even have the potential for morbidity. On the other, medical conditions also give rise to psychosocial problems in terms of the influence of social factors (such as job loss) on interactive human behavior (such as an inability to fulfill parental role). It is noteworthy, however, that although the use of the term "psychosocial" is widespread in the literature, its meaning is rarely explained, inference being that it may imply different things to different people. Even a quick glance at the relevant literature reveals this confusion. The more common confusion emanates from a lack of clarification of what may constitute psychosocial problems. Several studies investigate the presence of psychosocial problems in medical conditions, but they differ significantly in their meaning (Harada et al., 2002; Harter et al., 2004; Motamedi and Meador, 2003; Si et al., 2004).

This confusion about definition was noted in an investigation of the presence of psychosocial problems in primary care practice (Sheff et al., 1994). The authors noted that "Defining what constitutes a psychosocial problem in a physician visit is a surprisingly complex task. Most prevalence studies of psychosocial problems have addressed only psychiatric disorders, yet have documented very high rates, some as high as 50% to 75% of all primary care visits" (p. 393).

The goal of this study was to test a new taxonomy of psychosocial problems presented to family physicians (Sheff et al., 1994). Altogether 30 physicians participated in this investigation, but there was wide variability among the physicians in their interpretation of the same clinical vignettes as well as the patients in their respective practices. The conclusion was that physicians vary widely in their identification of psychosocial issues.

However, several investigators have resolved the problem of definition by interchangeably using the terms social and psychosocial (Deliege, 2001; Keefler et al., 2001). Deliege (2001) in her comprehensive report on the classification system of social problems also noted that although general practitioners and primary caregivers face a number of "psychosocial" problems in everyday practice, these problems are not always identified. However, specific tools are available for screening social problems in primary care settings (Corney, 1988; Piccinelli, 1997). Deliege (2001), in collaboration with general practitioners, reported on a study designed to test list of problems in three dimensions of well-being (physical, mental, and social). List of problems were generated by the WHO Department of Mental Health and discussed at an international symposium. They were then tested in the field. A conceptual framework was developed for social problems as follows:

1. Problems within the family
2. Problems of social integration
3. Socioeconomic problems and basic needs
4. Problems with social institutions
5. Problems of violence in society
6. Functional and social consequences of diseases
7. Other problems

This study showed that the use of this tool in the training of general practitioners drastically increased the identification of psychosocial problems, but only in the short run. In the long run, however, old habits tended to prevail.

The person-in-environment (PIE) classification system to measure social problems has made a major contribution to effectively assessing a whole range of social problems confronting an individual (Karls et al., 1997). The PIE is a four-factor system:

1. *Social Role Functioning Problems*—this factor describes a client or patient's problems in social role functioning, i.e., their severity and duration, and the client's ability to cope with them.
2. *Environmental Problems*—this factor describes problems in the environment that affect the client's functioning.
3. *Mental Health Problems*—this factor describes the patient's mental health issues.
4. *Physical Health Problems*—this factor describes the patient's mental and physical health issues.

Each major category has several subcategories. It is noteworthy that subcategories under Mental Health and Physical Health problems are based on Axis II and Axis III of DSM-IV, respectively. A numerical coding system enables the practitioner to have a shorthand for recording the results of PIE assessment.

Unfortunately, research or clinical literature on application of this instrument is almost absent. It is hard to assess its day-to-day use by practitioners. On the contrary, it is noteworthy that this instrument was translated into French and Japanese. The adoption of the PIE concepts and terminology into DSM-IV Axis IV further confirms its value. The pros and cons of the PIE system have received very limited attention (Karls et al., 1997).

Only one empirical report on its application was found (Keefler et al., 2001). This study investigated the effects of psychosocial problems on the length of stay in an acute care hospital. Using the PIE, data were collected from 160 patients: 78 in psychiatry and 82 in medical/surgical wards. Using regression analysis, Keefler et al. determined that the severity of the patients' psychosocial problems was a more significant predictor of length of stay than the diagnostic-related group (DRG) variables, which include medical diagnosis, basic demographics, and procedural information. Each DRG was associated with an average length of stay in hospital. A key finding was that a very high proportion of patients reported social role problems, mainly in their functioning as family members, workers, or students. These factors were more powerful predictors of length of stay than the severity of the medical problems. Although the authors found PIE to be a useful tool, they cautioned that the instrument was untested and there was some risk centered on interrater reliability.

Sheppard and colleagues (2005) conducted an update on the benefits of discharge planning. They reviewed 11 RCTs to determine the effectiveness of planning the discharge of patients from hospitals. The subjects included medical, surgical, and psychiatric patients. The findings were mixed. For example, one trial comparing a structured care pathway for patients recovering from a stroke reported significant rate of improvement compared with that of the control group. In contrast, two trials that reported satisfaction with discharge planning failed to attain statistically significant difference with patients who had routine discharge. The conclusion was that the impact of discharge planning on readmission rates, hospital length of stay, health outcomes, and cost was uncertain mainly because of different reported measures of outcome. However, the authors noted that even a small reduction in readmission rate, for example, brought about by discharge planning can result in very positive outcomes.

Reference was made earlier to the Axis IV of DSM-IV. This axis, known as the Psychosocial and Environmental Problems, may affect the diagnosis, treatment, and prognosis of mental disorders. The problems are grouped in the following categories:

- Problems with primary support group
- Problems related to the social environment
- Educational problems
- Occupational problems
- Housing problems
- Economic problems
- Problems with access to healthcare services
- Problems related to interaction with the legal system/crime

Examples are provided for each category but there are no firm guidelines, thus creating a certain amount of latitude for the clinician. The DSM-IV is very clear that most psychosocial and environmental problems are indicated on Axis IV.

According to Axis IV, a psychosocial or environmental problem may be a negative life event, an environmental difficulty or deficiency, a familial or other interpersonal stress, an inadequacy of social support or personal resources, or other problems related to the context in which a person's difficulties have developed. There are, however, no specific guidelines or instrument(s) to objectively assess the impact of these problems on the diagnosis, treatment, and prognosis of mental disorders. A more useful way of evaluating these social and environmental problems may be to determine the role of social factors in the genesis of a given psychiatric problem. Alternatively, they may be the consequence of a psychiatric disorder or, indeed, social factors may be the cause of much distress without any psychiatric consequences.

Report on Axis IV (psychosocial stressors in the last year, using DSM-III-R criteria) in the literature is indeed very sparse (Westermeyer and Specker, 1999). These authors reported on a study that compared 70 patients with substance-related disorder and eating disorder (SRD-ED) with 70 SRD patients only. The findings on the Axis IV were complex. SRD-ED patients had more advantageous social resources than SRD patients, including residence with family or friends, more education, higher socioeconomic status, and larger social networks. Perhaps contrary to expectation, SRD-ED patients showed a higher level of marriage and employment, and their coping levels were similar to those of SRD-only patients. The two groups showed strengths and weaknesses in different aspects of their social environment. These findings were unusual and could not be easily explained. They were certainly contrary to expectation as patients with comorbidity are expected to do less well than patients with a single disorder. Authors speculated that higher socioeconomic status of the SRD-ED patients compared with SRD-only patients may in part explain the finding. The authors recommended further research. In the absence of empirical research or clinical reports on Axis IV, the extent of its use in routine diagnostic investigation cannot be judged.

Axis V of DSM-IV is designed for reporting the clinician's judgment of the individual's overall level of functioning. Global Assessment of Functioning (GAF) Scale is used for this purpose. This scale is also of particular value in tracking the clinical progress of a patient in global terms. The GAF Scale cannot be used to assess impairment in functioning due to physical or environmental limitations. Axis V also proposes another scale, namely, Social and Occupational Functioning Assessment Scale (SOFAS), to track progress in rehabilitation independent of the severity of psychological symptoms. Hilsenroth and colleagues (2000) reported on the reliability and validity of DSM-IV Axis V. Their conclusion was that the GAF Scale was a valid measure of global psychopathology, and the SOFAS a measure of problems in social, occupational, and interpersonal functioning.

The GAF Scale has been used in various investigations. We provide a brief and selected review to show its usefulness when psychiatric and physical problems coexist for the simple reason that the rest of this volume is concerned with problems of chronic pain population where psychological and physical problems also coexist, and at times it is hard to decode which has the preeminence.

Bass and colleagues (2002) reported on a study that involved 900 patients referred to an outpatient liaison service. Assessments of functional capacity were measured by using the GAF Scale, and each patient was also assigned a psychiatric diagnosis using ICD-10 criteria. The most common reason for referral was somatic symptoms or pain (86%). Nearly 39% of patients had a concomitant physical disease, the most common being gastrointestinal (20%), cardiovascular (14%), neurological (11%), and respiratory (9%). Almost all patients were diagnosed with somatoform pain disorder, hypochondriasis, and unspecified somatoform disorders. Our subsequent discussion will show some of the difficulties associated with these diagnoses in chronic pain sufferers.

In fact, the authors were cognizant of the fact that managing patients with high level of disability, as many patients were in their sample, was problematic mainly because the focus was on serious mental illnesses in psychiatric treatment. They proposed specialized programs within psychiatry to specifically provide treatment for these type of patients with complex medical and psychiatric issues. In reality, many of these patients make their way into pain clinics, if and when available.

The commonest problems causing ongoing distress in this study population were physical health (28%), employment (20%), relationship with partner (14%), and recent loss (5%). The authors noted that one of the most striking finding was the high rate of functional impairment in these patients. The fact that one of three was not able to work was noteworthy. Nevertheless, these findings were consistent with high levels of functional impairment in patients with fibromyalgia and chronic fatigue syndrome. These findings have considerable significance for chronic pain sufferers.

Ruzickova and colleagues (2003) compared type 2 diabetic and bipolar disorder patients ($n = 26$) with only bipolar disorder patients ($n = 196$). This sample was obtained from the Maritime Bipolar Registry (Canada). Diabetic patients were older than nondiabetic patients. The diabetic group scored significantly higher on the GAF Scale ($p = 0.01$), were more often on disability, and had other medical complications. Unfortunately, this report did not give the details of their findings related to the GAF Scale. Nevertheless, the findings of this study support the notion that medical problems combined with psychiatric create more psychosocial problems. Again, this is relevant to any discussion of chronic pain patients, many of whom also suffer from some form of psychiatric disorders, mainly depression and anxiety.

Although there is ready recognition of the merit of incorporating psychosocial problems in the assessment and treatment of psychiatric and medically ill patients, the extent to which this kind of assessment is routinely carried out remains an open question. One would expect that in the practice of psychiatry, examination of the patient's environment and accompanying social problems would be of paramount importance. There is also a long tradition in psychiatry for doing so.

In our own work we have used the concept of social dislocation to assess the impact of chronic pain on the social environment of the patient (Roy, 2007). Within this perspective, a patient's social network is divided into three types: formal, semi-formal, and informal. The formal network includes medical services, insurance, workers compensation board, government agencies, and legal system. The semiformal includes the workplace, church, volunteer organizations, and family physician, and the informal network would consist of spouse/partners, children, parents, close friends, neighbors, and other intimates.

This model provides the clinician with a clear road map and enables her/him to organize a systematic review of the patient's social environment at the point of entry into the pain clinic. We shall demonstrate its application throughout this volume. At this point, we make a key observation that as the patient embarks on a career of chronicity, the shift in the social network is from the strong informal system to the formal system. The reason for this is obvious. As the patient's interaction with the medical world and other formal systems rises, there is almost a corresponding decline in interaction with the informal and semiformal systems. This particular approach combines two critical elements of the patient's environment: the presence of social stressors and the state of social support.

Unquestionably, some progress is evident even in our modest review in developing a meaningful taxonomy for social problems. Close scrutiny would reveal that basically they cover the same ground. Use of the PIE system, which holds much promise, does not appear to be widespread. All the efforts in family medicine to establish a common and systematic approach to investigate psychosocial problems have met with mixed results. The point still remains that without such taxonomy, identification of social problems remains somewhat a hit-and-miss proposition. This has serious implications for application of EBP to counter social problems that seem to be endemic to medical illness.

In the following section we explore the EBP literature to ascertain its application with psychosocial problems. The literature falls broadly into two categories (1) where the focus of intervention is identifiable social problems and (2) where the intervention is described as some form of psychosocial therapy.

Literature Review

Identifiable Social Problems and Social Interventions

A careful search of the Cochrane Library revealed a number of reports that fit the description of social intervention to redress identifiable social problems. Three of these reports address the issue of effective parenting to deal with behavioral problems in children (Barlow and Parsons, 2005; Coren and Barlow, 2005; Woolfenden et al., 2005). We summarize their key findings. Barlow and Parsons (2005) included five studies, all RCTs in their review that tested the effectiveness of group-based training programs for improving behavioral adjustment of 0–3 year old children. Their conclusion was that there was insufficient evidence to reach any firm conclusions. Long-term effectiveness was questionable. They recommended further research.

Woolfenden and colleagues (2005) examined the current evidence for the effectiveness of family and parenting intervention programs through a review of eight trials that met their criteria of RCTs. Their conclusion about these interventions was optimistic and they noted that family and parenting interventions were indeed capable of reducing time spent in institutions by juvenile delinquents. They speculated that these interventions may also reduce subsequent incarceration, but there were not enough data to fully support that conclusion.

The final review in this section was reported by Coren and Barlow (2005). They reviewed the RCT literature on the effectiveness of individual-based and/or group-based programs to improve psychosocial and developmental outcomes in teenage mothers. The results were obtained from four studies. These results showed improvement on mother–infant interaction, language development, parental attitudes, parental knowledge, maternal self-confidence, and maternal identity. On the contrary, because of the small number of studies, authors pointed to the limitations of their conclusions and urged further research.

Cochrane Reviews report on various issues that could broadly fit into the definition of psychosocial problems. These reports do not fit into any neat categories. They range from community interventions for reducing smoking (Secker-Walker et al., 2005) to the efficacy of supported housing for seriously mentally ill persons (Chilvers et al., 2005). This brief incursion into the Cochrane Library leaves no room for doubts that new and novel interventions are constantly being tried and reported for complex psychosocial problems.

A simple reality is that the literature on EBP of psychosocial problems is meager. The same can be said about social therapy, unless the definition is broadened to include therapies such as family therapy. A literature search (PsycINFO) on "EBP and psychosocial" produced only two relevant studies: (1) a report on the efficacy of psychoeducation for family members of psychotic patients (Murray-Swank and Dixon, 2004) and (2) a report on the utilization of daily journal club to address psychosocial issues in palliative care (Mazuryk et al., 2002). We present a brief description of these two innovative interventions and their effectiveness.

Murray-Swank's study reported that more than 30 randomized clinical trials demonstrated that psychoeducational programs for people with schizophrenia and bipolar disorder reduce relapse, improve symptomatic recovery, and enhance psychosocial and family outcomes. Furthermore, this review summarized findings or prominent psychoeducational programs. Mazuryk et al. reported in a different order. The authors described a unique daily journal club format used by their palliative care program and presented the results of a questionnaire sent to 24 family medicine residents and 20 palliative care fellows. The number of articles presented over 1 year was 252. Palliative care fellows showed a much higher level of satisfaction than did family medicine residents in areas of clinical applicability, acceptability of daily routine, and overall educational value. The increased emphasis on EBP in palliative care suggests that a journal club could be of great value. This article is valuable for another reason as it provides a clear tool for promoting EBP. This article also raises the old question of what may actually be termed "psychosocial." The journal program is undoubtedly a purely educational endeavor, and yet the literature search using the terms "EBP and psychosocial" produced this, albeit interesting, article. Does it really meet the definition of psychosocial?

A PsycINFO computer search on "social problems and EBP" produced ten results. Only two articles were empirically based. The first reported on the need for mediation in resolving divorce issues acknowledging that while mediation in the West had proved successful, it had to be culturally adapted to the needs of the Hong Kong Chinese population (Sullivan, 2005). The second article reported a review of interventions with antisocial behaviors of delinquent youth (Stern, 2004). Treatment–outcome research established that families were key agents for change for antisocial behaviors that included a whole host of social problems such as drug use, school failure, and depression, among the youth. This chapter provided a comprehensive review of the empirical literature on risk and protective factors, with attention to strong and modifiable determinants of antisocial behavior and delinquency. Family treatment approaches, which have proven effective, were emphasized.

Finally, in this section, we briefly review recent literature on the effectiveness of social therapy. It should be noted at the outset that there does not seem to be any consensus on what may or may not constitute social therapy. Any intervention that is nonmedical or not specifically addressing medical problems seems to come under the rubric of social therapy. One defines social therapy as a philosophically informed method that is uniquely focused on the creative capacity of groups of people to perform their own emotional growth (Holtzman and Mendez, 2003). Another posits that a certain type of group therapy that has its roots in mathematics is social therapy for group activity (Newman, 2003). This method of social therapy emphasizes the creative "unresolvability" to emotional growth. The definition of social therapy seems to be in the eye of the beholder.

A PsycINFO search on "social therapy" produced 163 results. Almost all articles were descriptive, as described earlier, and nonempirical, and thus outside the scope of this chapter. We provide a selected sample of the literature that reports on the efficacy of "social therapy." One study reported on the benefit of day care for dementia patients by implementing social therapy over inpatient care (Weyer et al., 2004). A cross-sectional study of 17 geriatric daycare facilities in eight towns and cities in Baden, Germany, examined the data for all 257 clients who received care on a given reference date. These clients were compared with an inpatient population of 15 randomly selected nursing homes and residential facilities. The average age of subjects in both groups was around 80 years. The results showed that moderate to severe dementia was equally distributed between the two groups. However, while the inpatient sector tended to place greater importance on basic care and treatment, daycare facilities focused primarily on measures of social therapy (e.g., group activities). They concluded that for a selected group of patients in day care, social therapy provided at least partial stress relief for family caregivers.

Another uncontrolled study, more a clinical report, related to the elderly suffering from Alzheimer's disease reported the benefit of music (social) therapy (Pollack and Namazi, 1992). In eight adults, this therapy implemented over 2 weeks indicated a 24% increase in social (interactional) behaviors.

We have provided a window into what may pass for social therapy which one might be inclined to think is the appropriate intervention(s) with social problems. In fact, this term engenders as much confusion as does the term psychosocial or even just social. The lack of consensus on the problems of definition is almost insurmountable. In fact, standard psychotherapeutic approaches can also fall under the rubric of social therapy. Our goal is to avoid terms in the rest of this volume that only create confusion and debate. We shall endeavor to identify the therapies as clearly as possible, and the same will hold true for problems.

As an illustration of that, we begin by a review of solution-focused therapy (SFT), which provides a powerful example of an interpersonal psychotherapy developed on the principles of brief therapy (de Shazer, 1988). The focus of SFT is in the here and now, and the underlying assumption is that we all have the power within ourselves to resolve our difficulties, albeit with some help. The model is very definitely predicated on the strength paradigm rather than on psychopathology. In his Preface to the book *Keys to Solution in Brief Therapy*, de Shazer (1985) stated: "This book describes a general view of solutions and how they work and of related specific procedures that have been developed during 15 years of doing and studying brief therapy." Ginerich (2000) operationally defined SFT as one or more of the following core components: (1) a search for presession change; (2) goal setting; (3) use of miracle question; (4) use of scaling questions; (5) a search for exceptions; (6) a consulting break; and (7) a message including compliments and tasks.

A major review on the efficacy of SFT was reported in 2000 (Ginerich, 2000). One rather striking observation was the use of SFT to address a very wide range of problems. First, we review the key findings of this review and, second, we conduct a further review of the more recent literature on the outcome of SFT. Ginerich's review, first and foremost, confirms the wide application of SFT to treat an impressive array of problems that include depression in college students, parenting skills, rehabilitation of orthopedic patients, recidivism in prison population, antisocial youths, couple problems, and problem drinking.

Ginerich classified 15 studies that met the inclusion criteria, which were based on the standards of outcome research established by APA, into three groups. This approach basically established a hierarchy of evidence for SFT. The first group, consisting of five papers, was judged to be "well-controlled" studies by virtue of their design. They were either randomized group design or "acceptable" single-case design. The second group, the "moderately controlled" studies consisting of four papers, focused on a specific problem. The final group, consisting of six papers, was judged "poorly controlled."

Ginerich's (2000) conclusions were cautious. The quality of design even for the well-controlled studies posed questions. Even these studies did not meet all the stringent criteria of outcome studies. One critical issue was the lack of studies that compared SFT with another type of psychotherapy. One study that did, produced equivalent outcome. Was the improvement attributable to SFT or general attention effects? Furthermore, because of the diverse study populations, Ginerich concluded that the efficacy of SFT could not be confirmed. Ginerich ends his article on an optimistic note. Efficacy of SFT is not an established fact. Yet, the studies taken together do provide preliminary support for SFT as an effective form of psychotherapy. The wide variety of populations and situations reported in these studies argue well for SFT. More carefully designed studies are called for. Ginerich's review included articles published up to 1999.

We revisit one of the studies reported by Ginerich in the "well-controlled" category that has relevance to the rest of this book. This study on a group of patients with orthopedic injuries evaluated the efficacy of SFT on the psychosocial adjustment and their return to work (Cockburn et al., 1997). This study involved 48 patients and their partners who were referred to a rehabilitation program following injuries for return to work by an orthopedic surgeon. These patients were first-time recipients of workers' compensation, who were not on prescription drugs, without any major medical problems, and with the spouse in full-time employment.

Subjects were randomly assigned to one of four groups. The treatment groups 1 and 3 received 6 weekly 1-hour program of SFT plus the routine rehabilitation program. It is noteworthy that treatment was administered by one of the authors and it followed a standard protocol. Control groups 2 and 4 received only the standard rehabilitation program.

Pretest data were collected for treatment group 1 and control group 2 using the Family Crisis Oriented Personal Evaluation Scales (F-COPES). Posttest data were collected from all four groups using the F-COPES and the Psychosocial Adjustment to Illness Scale–Self-Report (PAIS-SR). The results were impressive. Within

7 days of completion of treatment, 68% in the treatment group had returned to work compared with 4% in the control group. Thirty days after treatment the numbers increased to 92% and 47%, respectively.

Although the results were impressive and the design was relatively rigorous, the sample size was small. Nevertheless, the magnitude of change (return to work) was significant enough to demonstrate the efficacy of SFT. Questions can be raised about the specificity of the effects of SFT, but the data leave little doubt that SFT is an effective psychosocial intervention for injured patients with the goal of returning to work. However, an inescapable fact is that this study failed to meet the key criteria of APA Task Force of efficacy of treatment, namely, comparison with another treatment or placebo or pill, equivalent to an already established treatment in experiments with adequate sample size, or RCT, or a prescribed single-case study.

How much new evidence has emerged about the efficacy of SFT since 1999? Since 2000, PsycINFO revealed 32 studies on the efficacy of SFT. A vast majority of these studies did not meet some of the essential criteria of APA for outcome research. We report on a selected number of articles that at the very least used a control group. Wettersten and colleagues (2004) reported a study that compared brief interpersonal therapy (BIT) with solution-focused brief therapy (SFBT). Subjects ($n = 38$) for the BIT group were obtained from a previously published study and served as the comparison group. They were treated by 37 therapists. These subjects were clients at a university-based counseling center. The SFBT subjects ($n = 26$) also were drawn from clients treated at a university-based counseling center. These subjects were seen by 14 therapists. The authors acknowledged that a number of potential confounds prevented them from testing the relative merit of each intervention. This study compared the relationship between working alliance and outcome. The findings were intriguing. Working alliance, heavily emphasized in SFBT, was found not to be significantly related to the outcome for SFBT clients. On the contrary, the outcome for BIT clients was significantly related to working alliance. In general terms, the authors concluded that the results of this study suggested that SFBT could promote working alliance and that this alliance may play a different role in reducing psychological distress and promoting client satisfaction within the SFBT approach. The findings were tentative at best.

This study is fraught with methodological shortcomings. Apparently, limited information on the presenting problems of the BIT group was less than satisfactory. This also applied to the number of sessions per client. In both studies a huge number of therapists were involved. The therapists were at different levels of training. This study clearly failed to meet some very basic requirements of a controlled study, although it is one of the few studies that did compare SFT with another psychological intervention.

Another study tested the effectiveness of SFT against drug treatment for obsessive-compulsive disorder (Fan Ru et al., 2005). Sixty subjects with obsessive-compulsive disorder were randomly assigned to control group (paroxetine only, $n = 30$) and experimental group (paroxetine + SFT, $n = 30$). The treatment period was 10 weeks. The efficacy was tested using Yale–Brown Obsessive-Compulsive

Rating Scale (Y-BOCS) at the end of weeks 2, 4, 6, 8, and 10. The score for the experimental group was significantly lower on the Y-BOCS than that for the control group. The key finding was that SFT + paroxetine was significantly superior to paroxetine alone in the treatment of obsessive-compulsive disorder. This was a well-designed and well-executed study. The key finding for the efficacy of SFT is encouraging.

We report on one unique study that compared SFT with common factors therapy (CFT) conducted exclusively over the telephone (Rhee et al., 2005). Fifty-five subjects were recruited from a pool of callers to a suicide hotline, and were randomly assigned to a waiting list, SFT, and CFT. The results confirmed that the two therapy conditions were significantly more effective compared with the waiting list control (WLC). No significant differences emerged between the two treatment groups. Two more studies that included control groups reported on the efficacy of SFT: one was with cancer patients (Nairn, 2004) and the other with high-risk junior high school students (Newsome, 2004). Both these studies found support for SFT against "no treatment" control groups.

The results of outcome studies following Ginerich's (2000) excellent review, which included papers up to 1999, led to conclusions similar to his. Comparison of SFT with another psychosocial therapy remains more of an exception than the rule. Populations under study remain just as varied, and some of the methodological shortcomings that Ginerich identified can also be detected in more recent studies. The future researchers must focus on a narrower set of problems, compare SFT against other psychosocial therapies, and follow the standard procedure for randomized controlled studies with provision for at least a 2-year follow-up. Yet, the weight of the evidence minimally suggests that SFT is better than no therapy, and there is just the minimal of evidence to suggest that it may be superior to at least another psychotherapy method (Rhee et al., 2005). The jury is still out on the efficacy of SFT, when judged against the gold standard of treatment outcome measures, namely, RCTs and even single-case studies.

Summary

Our effort in this chapter has been twofold: (1) we identified the difficulties that are inherent in our attempt to establish a taxonomy of social problems that would make their way into daily practice and (2) we chose a very popular psychosocial intervention, the SFBT, that is widely used by psychotherapists to judge its effectiveness. The evidence we found is not strong, yet hopeful. Its wide use might suggest that practicing psychotherapists are perhaps not as diligent in searching for evidence of effectiveness as one ought to be. RCTs are perhaps too high a standard to expect to judge the efficacy of psychosocial interventions. Hence, the hierarchy of evidence is critically important to any discussion about the effectiveness of psychosocial interventions. The weight of the body of research, for instance, in relation to SFT may suggest that despite many of the shortcomings we have noted, this remains an effective intervention at least in the eyes of practitioners. They argue that as far as they are concerned it works and their clients benefit from it. If they are to wait for the right kind of evidence, only their clients will suffer.

Another point of note is that the effectiveness of any psychotherapeutic intervention cannot have the precision of drugs or surgical interventions. Psychotherapy does not threaten life, and has far less potential of doing harm than drugs or surgical interventions. This, however, is no reason for seeking evidence. The point is that even the most carefully manualized treatment such as cognitive behavioral therapy (CBT) cannot dispense with the human factor. Therapist variables have confounded researchers forever. Yet, the value of RCTs, the gold standard of outcome research, is unquestionable, and must remain the ultimate test for establishing efficacy for psychotherapeutic interventions. This is not to suggest that all other, perhaps less powerful, evidence should be disregarded.

References

Barlow, J. and Parsons, J. (2005) Group-based parent training programs for improving emotional and behavioral adjustment in 0–3 year old children. Cochrane Database Syst. Rev., Issue 4.

Bass, C., Bolton, J., and Wilkinson, P. (2002) Referrals to a liaison psychiatry out-patient clinic in a UK general hospital: a report on 900 cases. Acta Psychiatr. Scand., 105: 117–125.

Chambless, D. (1995) Training and dissemination of empirically validated psychological treatments; report and recommendations. Clin. Psychol., 48: 3–23.

Chambless, D., Baker, M., Baucom, D., et al. (1998) Update on empirically validated therapies, II. Clin. Psychol., 51: 3–16.

Chilvers, R., Macdonald, G., and Hayes, G. (2005) Supported housing for people with severe mental disorders. Cochrane Database Syst. Rev., Issue 4.

Cockburn, J., Thomas, F., and Cockburn, O. (1997) Solution-focused therapy and psychosocial adjustment to orthopedic rehabilitation in a work hardening program. J. Occup. Rehabil., 7: 97–106.

Coren, E. and Barlow, J. (2005) Individual and group-based parenting programs for improving psychosocial outcomes for teenage parents and their children. Cochrane Database Syst. Rev., Issue 4.

Corney, R. (1988) Development and use of a short self-rating instrument to screen for psychosocial disorders. J. R. Coll. Gen. Pract., 38: 263–266.

Deliege, D. (2001) A classification system of social problems: concepts and influences on GPs' registration of problems. Soc. Work Health Care, 34: 195–238.

de Shazer, S. (1985) Keys to Solution in Brief Therapy. New York, W. W. Norton.

de Shazer, S. (1988) Clues: Investigating Solutions in Brief Therapy. New York, W. W. Norton.

Diagnostic and Statistical Manual of Mental Disorders IV (1994) American Psychiatric Association.

Fan Ru, Y., Shaung Luo, Z., and Wen Feng, L. (2005) Comparative study of solution focused brief therapy combined with paroxetine in the treatment of obsessive-compulsive disorder. Chin. Ment. Health J., 19: 288–290.

Ginerich, W. (2000) Solution-focused brief therapy: a review of the outcome research. Fam. Process, 39: 477–499.

Harada, Y., Satoh, Y., Sakuma, Y., et al. (2002) Behavioral and developmental disorders among conduct disorder. Psychiatry Clin. Neurosci., 56: 621–625.

Harter, M., Hahn, D., Baumeister, H., et al. (2004) Comorbidity in patients with musculoskeletal and cardiovascular diseases: prevalence rates, diagnosis and consequences for rehabilitation. J. Public Health (Germany), 12: 162–167.

Hilsenroth, M., Ackerman, S., Blagys, M., et al. (2000) Reliability and validity of DSM-IV axis V. Am. J. Psychiatry, 157: 1858–1863.

Holtzman, L. and Mendez, R. (2003) Psychological Investigations: A Clinician's Guide to Social Therapy. New York, Brunner-Routledge.

Karls, J., Lowery, C., Mattaini, M., et al. (1997) The use of the PIE (PERSON-IN-ENVIRONMENT) system in social work education. J. Soc. Work Educ., 33: 49–59.

Keefler, J., Duder, S., and Lechman, C. (2001) Predicting length of stay in an acute care hospital: the role of psychosocial problems. Soc. Work Health Care, 33: 1–16.

Mazuryk, M., Daeninck, P., Neumann, C.M., and Bruera, E. (2002) Daily journal club: an education tool in palliative care. Palliat. Med., 16: 57–61.

Motamedi, G. and Meador, K. (2003) Epilepsy and cognition. Epilepsy Behav., 4(Suppl. 2): 25–38.

Murray-Swank, A. and Dixon, L. (2004) Family psychoeducation as an evidence-based practice. CNS Spectr., 9: 905–912.

Nairn, R. (2004) Improving coping with cancer using mastery enhancement therapy. Dissertation Abstracts International. Section B: The Science and Engineering 65(5-B): 2641.

Newman, F. (2003) Undecidable emotions (What is social therapy? And how is it revolutionary?) J. Constructive Psychol., 16: 215–232.

Newsome, W. (2004) Solution-focused brief therapy groupwork with at-risk junior high school students: enhancing the bottom line. Res. Soc. Work Pract., 5: 336–343.

Piccinelli, M. (1997) Test retest reliability of the social problem questionnaire in primary care in Italy. Soc. Psychiatry Psychiatr. Epidemiol., 32: 57–62.

Pollack, N. and Namazi, K. (1992) The effects of music participation on the social behavior of Alzheimer's disease patients. J Music Ther, 29: 54–67.

Rhee, W., Merbaum, M., Strube, M., et al. (2005) Efficacy of brief telephone psychotherapy with callers to a suicide hotline. Suicide Life Threat. Behav., 35: 317–328.

Rostila, I. and Piirainen, K. (2004) Evidence based practice in Finland. In: Thyer, B. and Kazi, M. (Eds.) International Perspectives on Evidence Based Practice in Social Work. British Association of Social Workers. UK.

Roy, R. (2007) Social dislocation and the chronic pain patient. In: Bond, M. (Ed.) Encyclopedia of Pain. Heidelberg, Springer.

Ruzickova, M., Slaney, C., Garnham, J., et al. (2003) Clinical features of bipolar disorder with and without co-morbid diabetes mellitus. Can. J. Psychiatry, 48: 458–461.

Sackett, D., Richardson, W., Rosenberg, W., et al. (1997) Evidence Based Medicine: How to Practice and Teach EBP. New York, Churchill-Livingston.

Secker-Walker, R., Gnich, W., Platt, S., and Lancaster, T. (2005) Community interventions for reducing smoking among adults. Cochrane Database Syst. Rev., Issue 4.

Sheff, R., Rand, W., Paterson, J., et al. (1994) Psychosocial problems in primary care pilot study of a new taxonomy. J. Fam. Pract., 38: 393–403.

Sheldon, B. (2001) The validity of evidence based practice in social work: a reply to Stephen Webb. Br. J. Soc. Work, 31: 801–809.

Sheppard, S., Parkes, J., McClaran, J., and Phillips, C. (2005) Discharge planning from hospital to home. Cochrane Database Syst. Rev., Issue 4.

Si, J., Wang, L., and Chen, S. (2004) Irritable bowel syndrome consulters in Zhejiang province: the symptoms pattern, pre-dominant bowel habit sub-groups and quality of life. World J. Gastroenterol., 10: 1059–1064.

Smith, D. (Ed.) (2004) Social Work and Evidence Based Practice. London, Jessica Kingsley Publishers.

Stern, S. (2004) Evidence-based practice with anti-social and delinquent youth. In: Briggs, H. and Rzepnicki, T. (Eds.) Using Evidence in Social Work Practice: Behavioral Perspectives (pp. 104–127). Chicago, IL, Lyceum Books, Inc.

Sullivan, P. (2005) Culture, divorce, and family mediation in Hong Kong. Fam. Court Rev., 43: 109–123.

Thyer, B. (2004) Evidence based practice in the United States. In: Thyer, B. and Kazi, M. (Eds.) International Perspectives on Evidence-Based Practice in Social Work. British Association of Social Workers. UK.

Thyer, B. and Kazi, M. (2004) An overview of evidence based practice in social work. In: Thyer, B. and Kazi, M. (Eds.) International Perspectives on Evidence-Based Practice in Social Work. British Association of Social Workers. UK.

Webb, S. (2001) Some consideration on the validity of evidence based practice in social work. Br. J. Soc. Work, 31: 57–79.

Westermeyer, J. and Specker, S. (1999) Social resources a social function in co-morbid eating and substance disorder: a matched-pairs study. Am. J. Addict., 8: 332–336.

Wettersten, K., Lichtenberg, J., and Mallinckordt, B. (2004) Associations between working alliance and outcome in solution-focused brief therapy and brief interpersonal therapy. Psychother. Res., 15: 35–43.

Weyer, S., Schaufele, M., Schrag, A., and Zimber, A. (2004) Dementia disorders, behavior problems and care of clients in geriatric day care compared to residents in home for the elderly: a cross-sectional study in eight communities in Baden. Psychiatr. Prax., 17: 339–345.

Woolfenden, S., William, K., and Peat, J. (2005) Family and parenting interventions in children and adolescents with conduct disorder and delinquency aged 10–17. Cochrane Database Syst. Rev., Issue 4.

Chapter 2
Psychosocial Problems and the Chronic Pain Sufferer

An Evidential Perspective on Social Dislocation

Chronic illness, and indeed chronic pain, has the potential to turn a patient's life upside down. Much of what is of value is either compromised or lost. A person derives one's sense of self from what one does. Social roles are at the very center of one's identity. It is the loss of valued social roles and interpersonal relations resulting in massive social dislocation that calls for a redefinition of self, a path fraught with struggle and disappointment. Bannerjee (2003) noted that unlike medical and psychological problems, social problems associated with chronic pain are rarely addressed in the literature on chronic pain treatment. However, the emotional cost associated with not performing daily activities for patients with rheumatoid arthritis (RA) has been noted in the literature (Hommel et al., 2004), as has the fact that these patients often experienced significant deficits across a number of life domains, including work (Katz, 1995), household activities (Allaire et al., 1991), and service activities (Cornelissen et al., 1988).

Social dislocation is also observable in the chronic pain patients attending a pain clinic, among others, in the three domains: work, family relations, and social relations. This dislocation frequently results in social isolation. To demonstrate this consequence, first, we narrate the story of John and, second, we provide a selected literature review of the problems that ultimately overwhelm John.

John, in his early thirties, was injured in a work-related accident. He was a skilled construction worker, very knowledgeable in the field of commercial construction. His skills were much sought after. He was married with a small baby. His wife worked and between the two of them they had a substantial income. John's parents were alive, and he maintained a very close relationship with them. He was a churchgoer, had an extensive network of friends, and belonged to a number of social organizations. Just before the accident, his relationship with his employer soured. He had several thousand dollars worth of tools stolen at a building site, but the employer refused any liability. Otherwise, he had enjoyed a very fruitful working relationship with this person.

The accident did not seem very serious. Trying to lift some material, he fell and bruised his buttocks and low back. He was off for a few days and then returned to work, hoping to complete his assignment. It did not take long for John to realize that he was having difficulty even doing simple tasks as his pain worsened. He took some time off, and thus began his journey through the healthcare system. Extensive

R. Roy, *Psychosocial Interventions for Chronic Pain*,
DOI: 10.1007/978-0-387-76296-8_2 © Springer Science+Business Media, LLC 2008

radiological, orthopedic, and neurological investigations failed to explain his then persistent and almost unbearable pain, about which he was skeptical. He applied for workers' compensation. His employer denied any culpability. Compensation was denied. Thus began John's not so slow descent into poverty and chronicity.

His assumptive world was beginning to collapse all around him. He was already in conflict with three formal systems: the medical board, the employer, and the compensation board. His family situation worsened. There was a measurable change in his roles and attitudes. Sexual activities came to a halt. He assumed the role of the baby minder as they could no longer afford day care. The role of the homemaker was thrust upon him. He enjoyed taking care of the baby but resented the rest. This family had no savings and they could no longer afford their mortgage payment. They sold their home and moved in with his wife Joan's family. His pain continued unabated, his mood soured, and the level of tension between him and Joan was palpable. John described his life as "living a nightmare."

In the meantime, his search for a medical cure gained pace. The family outings disappeared and his social activities came to a virtual halt. All this happened in a matter of 6 months. He became obsessed with his misfortune. He was full of shame and guilt over his failure to provide for his family, pain remained a mystery, and he lost all sense of enjoyment. Loss of self-esteem combined with hopelessness and helplessness were the dominant emotions. Not a single aspect of his life remained untouched by pain. Almost all his sources of social support dried up. The genesis of all of this was a seemingly minor work-related accident. It was at this point that his family physician referred him to a pain clinic. In the following section we analyze the extent of John's social dislocation by identifying those areas and by an examination of the pertinent literature. We discuss the problems not uncommonly encountered by chronic pain patients (certainly faced by John) that we consider to be of relevance. These problems are also reported in the literature in varying depths.

Chronic Pain and Unemployment

First and foremost, John lost his work and his means of livelihood. In our culture work occupies a unique position. The very first question we are often asked when meeting someone new in a social situation is, "What do you do?" It is a source of prestige, and a way of judging our social pecking order. Beyond that, it is a means of making a living, and much of our sense of who and what we are seem to be tied to what we do. Work is also a social organization. Friendships and camaraderie are often formed in our workplace. For John, losing employment had major consequences. We explore some of those consequences. Unemployment caused by accidents and health problems carries the added burden of coping with poor health and the job. Chronic pain and unemployment produce rather similar psychological and emotional responses (Roy, 2007). Both generate family conflict, social isolation, and loss of roles. Unemployment also contributes to family violence, suicide, family crisis, and health problems (Roy, 2001).

A major Canadian study involving 14,313 subjects revealed far-reaching effects of unemployment (D'Arcy and Siddique, 1987). Significant differences emerged between the employed and the unemployed: the unemployed showing a higher level of distress, short-term and long-term disabilities, numerous health problems, and greater utilization of health services. Interaction effects of socioeconomic status and demographics showed an association between employment status and emotional health. The blue-collar workers were more prone to physical illness in contrast to white-collar workers, who seemed more prone to emotional distress. Low-income unemployed, who were the principal wage earners, were the most psychologically distressed group. An inescapable truth is that the pain clinic population is well represented by the last group. It serves as a double-edged sword, because insufficient education is a known barrier to returning to work among individuals suffering from musculoskeletal disorders. Fear of layoff and unemployment is common in workers with low-back strain injuries, resulting in lost time. Recent studies, more or less, confirm the psychological and social ill effects of unemployment (Classen et al., 1993; Eales, 1998; Hall and Johnson, 1998).

The actual number of studies investigating unemployment in the chronic pain population remains few. A high rate of unemployment was reported among chronic pain patients in a comparative study of headache and back pain patients (Stang et al., 1998). The sample consisted of 662 subjects with headache and 1024 with back pain. Over the study period of 3 years, 13% of headache and 18% back pain subjects remained unemployed because of their pain conditions. Among the employable, 12% were unemployed. Grading of chronic pain emerged as a significant factor in predicting unemployment and disability, and the highest level of chronic pain predictably showed the highest levels of affective distress. Unemployment was strongly associated with pain levels, which is true for any pain clinic population who tend to suffer high levels of pain.

A more recent study also confirmed these results (James et al., 2005). Subjects were 141 adults with arthritis. The results showed that subjects with greater pain disability experienced, among other things, higher unemployment. Having a job to return to also predicts a better outcome for chronic pain sufferers (Loomis, 2005). However, it is noteworthy that many chronic pain patients do not recover sufficiently to return to work, irrespective of a job to return to. Another study compared patients with depression ($n = 173$) with a group with arthritis ($n = 87$) and found that at the 6-month follow-up persons with depression had significantly more unemployment than the group with arthritis (Lerner et al., 2004).

Depression or depressive symptoms is nevertheless a common comorbid condition of chronic pain in a significant proportion of chronic pain patients (Roy, 2001). Averill and colleagues (1996) investigated the impact of unemployment on depression in 300 patients randomly selected from 1000 patients referred to a pain clinic. A remarkable 67% were unemployed. Unequivocal support was found for an association between unemployment and increased depressive symptoms.

Jackson et al. (1998) studied the complex nature of the effects of unemployment in a group of 83 chronic pain patients and 88 healthy controls. After controlling for the length of current unemployment and number of pain sites, several psychosocial measures, such as purposeful time use, perceived financial security, and social support from formal sources, emerged as the most significant predictors of emotional distress in both the groups. This is one of a very few studies that directly addressed the consequences of chronic pain and unemployment and their power to predict emotional distress. A recent study also showed that in a return-to-work program for patients with chronic low-back pain (CLBP), those who failed either to return to work or engage in voluntary activities had higher scores on somatic anxiety and depression and longer duration of unemployment (Watson et al., 2004). Turner and Turner (2004) in an investigation of the joint effects of unemployment and physical disability, however, found that there was no overlap in their psychological impact, the two stressors representing cumulative, and even synergistic, adversity. Persons with disabilities were five times more likely than healthy controls to be unemployed. However, this difference accounted for only about 30% of the elevations in depression for the disabled group compared with the healthy subjects. These findings are counterintuitive and require further replication.

The fact, however, remains that the potential effects of chronic pain and unemployment combined can only add to the psychosocial distress of our patients. They share many common consequences such as family conflict, depression, social isolation, loss of roles, and somatization. Unemployment has added risks for suicide, family violence, and often financial problems. To return to John, if he had to contend only with his pain, but somehow managed to continue to work, the degree of social dislocation and psychosocial distress he experienced would have been far less drastic. Inability to work had very far-reaching consequences for John.

Family Relations

John's little family came apart at the seams. Not all families with chronic pain meet with such drastic fate, but changes in the family system and its capacity to adapt to a chronic pain sufferer in its midst can and does have far-reaching consequences. In this section, we consider the changes that occur in a family system because of the chronic pain. This literature is well established, but one fact worthy of reiteration is that in the past 5 or more years research on family and chronic pain has come to a virtual halt (Roy, 2006).

Research is indeed rich and diverse in the field of chronic pain and family function. Although the findings can be contradictory at times, the overall consensus is that families are somewhat adversely affected by chronic pain. Apart from the obvious impact on family roles and communication, for example, there is also considerable evidence to suggest the vulnerability of the well partner (especially female partners) to fall prey to psychological distress and depression. Given the intensity of change that chronic pain can induce in a family functioning, this is hardly surprising. John's case attests to this fact. His wife, Joan, would require an extraordinary level of resilience to remain immune to the changes in their fortune.

Family roles, communication, capability for free expression of feelings, family organization, and family cohesion all come under attack. We begin by taking a broad view of the overall impact of chronic pain conditions on family function. One American study employed the survey method to assess the social and personal impact of headache in a community sample of headache sufferers in Kentucky (Kryst and Scherl, 1994). A total of 647 subjects were assessed for serious headache. The 12-month period of prevalence for all serious headache was 13.4%. Majority of these people (73.6%) reported that headache had negatively affected at least one aspect of their lifestyle. Of these, 20% of males and 62% of females reported negative impact on their family relations. Efficiency at work, attending social events, capacity for planning ahead, relations with friends, and self-image are an impressive list of problems reported by a significant proportion of the headache sufferers. It must be obvious from the list of problems that many aspects of family life were influenced by headaches.

In a nationwide survey of 400 persons, Smith (1998) identified 350 migraine sufferers, of whom 269 were females and 81 males. This is a study of some significance as it explored many aspects of family life. A majority of 61% reported that their headache had a significant impact on their families. Families were generally sympathetic or understanding of the member with headache. Yet, headache delayed or postponed household duties for 79% of the respondents, and 64% reported that activities with children and spouses were adversely affected.

The household activities delayed or postponed included for 81% housecleaning and yard work, 79% laundry and shopping, 76% cooking, 69% activities with spouse, 62% activities with children, and 18% staying in bed. One striking finding was that 61% of the subjects were compromised in their care of children under 12 years. This included 61% canceling plans for playing, helping with homework, or spending together. An amazing 66% of the children learned to keep quiet, 25% were confused, and another 17% were hostile. A large number of younger children had their normal childhood relations and activities interrupted.

For the older children between the ages of 12 and 17 years, 87% stopped playing music or engaged in noisy activities, 61% stopped asking questions or for help with homework, 42% stopped inviting friends home, and 34% stopped visiting friends. However, 87% of the children over the age of 12 showed more understanding about the pain and 42% were even helpful. Finally, 25% of the migraine sufferers reported that their pain had a negative effect on their partner or spousal relationship. For a full 24% of the respondents, frequency and/or quality of sexual relationship deteriorated. Despite all these difficulties, only 5% reported divorce, and another 5% cited headache as a cause for separation from partner. Another study investigated the effects of complex regional pain syndrome (CRPS) on employment status, time allocation, the need for additional domestic help, and out-of-pocket expenses in 50 Dutch patients and 43 spouses (Kemler and Furnee, 2002). The results were compared with the Dutch population. In households with male patients, full-time employment decreased by 47%, which caused a decrease in income to the tune of $4000.00. The income loss for household with female patients was $2000.00. Compared with the Dutch population, patients spent less time on paid employment, and spent more time in household activities. Spouses were forced to spend time doing domestic chores leaving less time for personal needs and recreation. Loss of income and reallocation of roles were the two clear outcomes. A number of survey-type studies have reported, in general terms, on the impact of chronic pain drawing similar conclusions that family activities and relationships are altered and affected for the worse (Roy, 2006).

The overall picture is bleak. Migraine, albeit a debilitating, is an episodic disease. Most patients between the bouts can and do function at some level. This last study is indicative of the potential of this disease to inflict measurable damage on almost all aspects of family life. Chronic pain patients we generally encounter in pain clinics tend to be disabled to various degrees and are not very functional. Their pains are persistent and often in the severe range. Common sense dictates that their family life will be seriously compromised. The average age, early to mid-forties, of a chronic pain sufferer is also an important factor. Life transition issues are critical in this stage of life (Thomas and Roy, 1999). Children leaving home, work issues, health problems, and identity crisis are not uncommon during this phase. The added burden of chronic pain only complicates the picture.

We now review a few selected studies that actually measured family functioning to assess the impact of chronic pain on family life. We take into account only more recent studies that reported on systemic changes in the family because of chronic pain. Much of this literature is somewhat dated as investigations into the family function from a systemic perspective of chronic pain patients have come to a virtual halt (Roy, 2006).

Two measures of family functioning, namely, the Family Environment Scale (FES) and Family Adaptability and Cohesion Scale (FACES III, Couple Version), have been used with the chronic pain population. In broad terms, both these measures point that chronic pain is capable of much disruption in family life. Five studies used the FES (Kopp et al., 1995; Naidoo and Pillay, 1994; Nicassio and Radojevic 1993; Nicassio et al., 1995; Romano et al., 1997). One of the unresolved problems is that even with similar populations, different studies found different outcomes. This makes generalization difficult beyond the obvious that chronic pain families function less effectively than healthy ones.

Kopp and colleagues (1995) investigated the impact of chronic pain in a group of mothers with headache and back pain and a control group. No significant differences were found between the clinical and the control group on 6 of the 10 subscales of FES: cohesion, conflict, independence, achievement orientation, intellectual orientation, and control. However, they differed from normal families in expressiveness, active recreational orientation, and moral-religious orientation. The clinical families were more deficient in expressing feelings, less spontaneous, and less able to express criticism or annoyance than the controls. Clinical families were also less active in their free time than the healthy controls. In general terms, although on most of the measures of FES the clinical and control groups were similar, there were some important differences.

On the contrary, Naidoo and Pillay (1994) in a comparison of 15 women with low-back patients and a control group found significant differences on the FES between the two groups on cohesion, conflict, independence, and organization. These findings represent a significant departure from Kopp's. Romano and colleagues

(1997) also used five subscales of FES with 50 chronic pain patients and controls. Pain patients were found wanting in the area of cohesion, but were similar on the rest of the measures. The two groups were more similar than different. These three studies taken together do suggest that family functioning of chronic pain families based on FES is somewhat compromised, but the areas of compromise vary considerably between the studies.

Nicassio and Radojevic (1993) demonstrated how low family cohesion on the FES in a group of patients with fibromyalgia contributed to psychological disturbance, and high systems maintenance, control, and low independence contributed to pain in patients with RA and fibromyalgia. In a subsequent study, Nicassio and colleagues (1995) further explored the significance of the family cohesion subscale of the FES and found that in a group of patients with fibromyalgia, family cohesion contributed an equal amount of variability to depression as that contributed by pain, and was a highly significant predictor of depression in this population. This study was a refined analysis of a particular aspect of family functioning and its clinical significance.

The FACES III (Couple Version) was used in a study of family functioning of 51 consecutive patients referred to an urban pain clinic located in a teaching hospital (Roy and Thomas, 1989). On the FACES, these families performed in the middle to extreme ranges, suggesting moderate to extreme difficulties, respectively. Family adaptability (to a chronic pain patient) posed a serious challenge to these families. Family cohesion, however, was less of a problem. Family connectedness was maintained somewhat tentatively by the well spouse, who assumed the task of keeping the family together. Another study using the FACES reported very different results. In their comparison of 117 headache patients with a control group, they failed to find significant differences on cohesion, protectiveness, adaptability, and satisfaction (Basolo-Kunzer et al., 1991).

The findings of many of these studies remain irreconcilable. Methodological issues could probably explain much of the confusion. Yet, the collective findings point that chronic pain is capable of disrupting family function in several ways. The survey type studies, on the contrary, provide considerable support for ongoing family difficulties encountered by families with a chronic pain patient in their midst. Overall, the power of the evidence is that dislocation in family relations brought on by chronic pain is not uncommon.

Social Support

Research literature is rich in detailing the benefits of social support or the price of inadequate social support. It is rather silent on the question of loss of or reduction in social support as a consequence of chronic illness. One known consequence of chronic pain on the well spouse is distress and even depression. It is reasonable to assume that depression in one partner and chronic pain in the other cannot maintain whatever the level of mutual support they had at the premorbid level. It is also a matter of common sense that social and recreational activities tend to decline for our patients. In other words, a price commonly paid by chronic pain sufferers is social isolation and withdrawal. For many of our patients, the collapse of their social world combined with stressful family situation is their daily reality. Research findings into the collapse or shrinkage of their social world remain somewhat indirect. However, research on the significance of social support for chronic pain sufferers is extensive. Reviews of that body of literature leave little doubt. Most of these studies tend to confirm an association between the lack of social support and the severity of pain (Roy, 2001, 2006). We provide a selected review of the most recent literature on the role of social support in the mitigation of pain.

One study that provides partial answer to the question of the effects of poor and persistent social support over a prolonged period was a prospective study involving 78 patients with RA whose long-term functional ability and social support were assessed at 1-year, 3-year, and 5-year intervals (Evers et al., 2003). Social support in the past 6 months was measured along two dimensions: the quantitative aspect such as the size of social network and the qualitative aspect such as the availability of emotional and instrumental support. The study was designed to investigate the long-term effects of pain-avoidance behavior and social support in coping with pain of RA. The results were unequivocal in terms of the value of social support. Poor social support consistently predicted a less unfavorable course of functional disability and pain at the 3-year and 5-year follow-ups and these effects occurred irrespective of personality characteristics of neuroticism and extroversion, clinical status, and use of medications affirming the power of social support. In other words, the power of social support to influence overall function and pain levels was found to be significantly influenced by the level of social support. An inference that can be drawn from this study is that over time inadequate social support for chronic pain sufferers does not seem to improve.

A more recent study confirmed the significance of social support in a comparative investigation of several chronic pain disorders and found that clinically defined chronic widespread pain and fibromyalgia patients showed more severe impairment of health status than the no pain controls and chronic widespread pain with a stricter definition (Bergman, 2005). Factors such as lower socioeconomic status, compromised housing, lower education, and lack of social support were associated with the more impaired groups. The author noted that the background variables were important to attend to in the understanding and management of chronic widespread pain and fibromyalgia.

The role of social support in coping with daily pain was reported in a unique study by Holtzman and associates (2004). Two hundred subjects with RA completed a number of questionnaires including a daily diary of pain levels, satisfaction or dissatisfaction with social support from the intimates and others, which included spouse, brother or sister, children, parent and parent-in-law, other relative, friend, neighbor, someone at work, or someone else. This study investigated the value of social support from the perspective of the role of social support in enhancing cognitive coping with pain associated with RA.

Social support was found to contribute to the development of coping strategies, and the effectiveness of these strategies. Furthermore, social support and coping were found to be inextricably linked. Satisfaction with support was linked to higher use of cognitive reframing, emotional expression, and problem solving. Social support, in addition, was a predictor of the effectiveness, with which patients were able to employ the use of stoic distancing to cope with their pain. The value of this study is that it demonstrated one of the mechanisms that underlie social support that went considerably beyond the commonsense perspective. Cognitive restructuring resulting in better coping with pain as a direct result of positive social support is a most encouraging development. The findings of this study add considerably to the commonly acknowledged buffer model of social support. However, another study on the role of social support in a group of 93 chronic pain patients failed to find evidence of the buffering role of social support (Beugnot, 2002). Buffering role of social support is well established in the chronic pain literature and, indeed, social support may operate in complex ways with more than a single mechanism explaining its effectiveness.

The final study we present was conducted with eight chronic pelvic pain (CPP) sufferers to investigate the helpful and unhelpful social support from their partners, families, friends, acquaintances, doctors, nurses, and other women with CPP (Warwick et al., 2004). A case study approach was used. This was a detailed investigation of the benefits of social support from a whole range of sources. Participants in this study valued emotional, informational, and tangible support from all members of the network. Given the nature of this study, it is not possible to aggregate the results. Nevertheless, this particular approach to investigating social support illuminates who may or may not be a source of effective social support with what kind of problems.

This brief review of the most recent literature failed to answer one key question: Does informal social support (partners and other intimates) tend to decline with advancing chronicity for pain sufferers with corresponding increase in formal support (hospitals, legal systems, workers' compensation board, etc.)? The actual value of social support was confirmed and reconfirmed. At a theoretical level, buffering role of social support was challenged, and an alternative in the way of cognitive coping was offered. More than one mechanism might explain the effectiveness of social support for moderating pain and promote healthy behavior. However, the power of social support to facilitate effective coping with chronic pain is undeniable.

Other Measures of Social Dislocation

Social dislocation of varying degree is easily observed in chronic pain sufferers attending a pain clinic. Sickness Impact Profile (SIP) (Bergner et al., 1981) and the West Haven–Yale Multidimensional Pain Inventory (WHYMPI) (Kerns et al., 1985) have been extensively used to assess the degree of psychosocial dislocation in the chronic pain population. Suffice it say that the studies utilizing these instruments have demonstrated repeatedly the extent of psychosocial problems encountered by chronic pain sufferers. These instruments while overlapping in some aspects also focus on somewhat different aspects of a patient's environment, but broadly, they cover the important aspects of a patient's psychosocial world.

WHYMPI is a brief self-administered inventory that is used for multidimensional assessment of chronic pain. The scales measure severity and interference of pain, as well as individual responses to pain and impact on daily activities. The scale has three sections containing several subscales. The first section of this inventory is relevant to our discussion as it investigates the pain interference in the performance of day-to-day activities, ability to work, enjoyment derived from social and recreational activities, and changes in these activities. In short, WHYMPI creates a comprehensive social profile of chronic pain sufferers showing the level of social dislocation. In terms of the validity of WHYMPI, the pain severity and interference dimension correlated with McGill Pain Questionnaire. The activity level, which is another dimension of WHYMPI, investigates the level of activities and thus is an indicator of not just the functional aspects, but also the patient's connectedness with the social world, such as visiting friends or relatives or going to movies or playing cards. Although this measure is not conventionally used to measure social isolation, it does give a picture of the patient's connectedness with the world outside. Since its introduction, this inventory has been extensively used, and is a reliable way of investigating the social aspects of a patient's life which have been affected by chronic pain.

SIP is a 136-item inventory designed to assess 12 dimensions of functioning, which includes mobility, work, household management, social interactions, and recreational pursuits (Bergner et al., 1981). The dimensions are combined to form Physical, Psychosocial, other, and an Overall Disability scales. Follick et al. (1985) have provided evidence for this measure's construct validity in chronic pain samples. They investigated 107 patients with CLBP. They found that SIP supported the validity associated with chronic pain. Patients suffering from CLBP showed significant impairment in physical health, psychosocial well-being, recreational activities, and work. The most affected area was work, but recreation, social interaction, and home management, among other factors, were also significantly affected. Compared with patients with RA patients, CLBP patients experienced very similar levels of impairment. Notably, CLBP patients experienced far greater disruption in the psychosocial arena. They found that SIP was well suited for the assessment of patients with chronic pain. SIP helped establish the extent of social and psychological distress experienced by chronic pain sufferers. Over the years, SIP has found favor with researchers in chronic pain and has been extensively used in research.

Summary

It is hard to establish the actual extent to which social problems are encountered by chronic pain sufferers. Prevalence and incidence of the problems we have discussed in this chapter are not altogether clear. Inventories such as WHYMPI and SIP can generate that information, but they have not been used solely for that purpose. We, in this chapter, attempted to explore three critical aspects of a patient's social environment: work, family, and social support. Despite some contradictory data, the evidence is powerful enough to suggest that family disruption due to chronic pain is relatively common. Spousal distress and even depression which we did not review, well documented in pain literature, is also a significant contributor to the overall disruption.

Job loss, which for many patients translates into loss of income, has far-reaching consequences for the patient and family, and has the potential of being a catastrophic event. We reviewed the consequences of job loss, and as was evident in the story of John the effects were devastating for him and his family. Again, it will be a fair observation that the consequences of job loss for our patients remain underinvestigated. Finally, we examined the role of social support and the consequences of poor support. We were unable to find clear evidence for the observed phenomenon that progression into chronicity for our patients brings about a shift in their support system—from informal to formal. Job combined with disruption of family equilibrium and loss of social support sets off a chain of events that may be deemed wholly undesirable, causing high level of distress in our patients. These patients tend to be at the far end of nonresponders to the usual pain management. By definition, they are a disadvantaged group. By the time they arrive at a pain clinic, they are not only confronted with pain that remains often impervious to treatment, but they also face challenges on many psychosocial fronts.

References

Allaire, S., Meehan, R., and Anderson, J. (1991) The impact of rheumatoid arthritis on the household work performance of women. Arthritis Rheum., 34: 669–678.

Averill, P., Novy, D., Nelson, D.E., et al. (1996) Correlates of depression in chronic pain patients: a comprehensive examination. Pain, 65: 93–100.

Bannerjee, S. (2003) The role of problem-solving in the adaptation of women to chronic pain. Dissertation Abstracts International. Section B: The Sciences and Engineering, 63(9B): 4360.

Basolo-Kunzer, M., Diamond, S., and Reed, J. (1991) Chronic headache patients' marital and family adjustment. Issues Ment. Health Nurs., 12: 133–148.

Bergner, M., Bobbitt, R., Carter, W., et al. (1981) The sickness impact profile: development and final revision of a health measure. Med. Care, 19: 787–805.

Bergman, S. (2005) Psychosocial aspects of chronic widespread pain and fibromyalgia. Disabil. Rehabil., 27: 675–683.

Beugnot, S. (2002) Pain beliefs, coping, and social support as predictors of physical and psychological adjustment in chronic pain beliefs. Dissertation Abstracts International. Section B: The Science and Engineering, 63(4B): 2049.

Classen, B., Bjorndal, A., and Hjort, P. (1993) Health and unemployment in a two year follow-up of long term unemployed. J. Epidemiol. Community Health, 47: 14–18.

Cornelissen, P., Rasker, J., and Valkenburg, H. (1988) The arthritis sufferer and the community: a comparison of arthritis sufferers in rural and urban areas. Ann. Rheum. Dis., 47: 150–156.

D'Arcy, C. and Siddique, C. (1987) Unemployment and health: an analysis of Canada health survey. Int. J. Health Serv., 15: 609–635.

Eales, M. (1998) Depression and anxiety in unemployed men. Psychol. Med., 18: 935–945.

Evers, A., Kraaimatt, F., Geene, R., et al. (2003) Pain coping and social support as predictors of long-term functional disability and pain in early rheumatoid arthritis. Behav. Res. Ther., 41: 1295–1310.

Follick, M., Smith, T., and Ahern, D. (1985) The sickness impact profile: a global measure of disability in chronic low-back pain. Pain, 21: 67–76.

Hall, E. and Johnson, L. (1998) Depression in unemployed Swedish women. Soc. Sci. Med., 27: 134–135.

Hommel, K., Wagner, J., Chaney, J., et al. (2004) Perceived importance of activities of daily living and arthritis helplessness in rheumatoid arthritis. J. Psychosom. Res., 57: 159–164.

Holtzman, S., Newth, S., and Delongis, A. (2004) The role of social support in coping with daily pain among patients with arthritis. J. Health Psychol., 9: 677–695.

Jackson, T., Lezzi, A., Lafraniere, K., et al. (1998) Relations of employment status to emotional distress among chronic pain patients: a path analysis. Clin. J. Pain, 14: 55–60.

James, N., Miller, C., Brown, K., and Weaver, M. (2005) Pain disability among older adults with arthritis. J. Aging Health, 17: 56–69.

Katz, P. (1995) The impact of rheumatoid arthritis on the life activities. Arthritis Care Res., 8: 272–278.

Kemler, M. and Furnee, C. (2002) The impact of chronic pain on life in the household. J. Pain Symptom Manage., 23: 433–441.

Kerns, R., Turk, D., and Rudy, T. (1985) The West-Haven-Yale Multidimensional Pain Inventory. Pain, 23: 345–356.

Kopp, M., Richter, R., Prisca, J., et al. (1995) Differences in family functioning between patients with chronic headache and patients with chronic low-back pain. Pain, 63: 219–224.

Kryst, S. and Scherl, E. (1994) A population based survey of the social and personal impact of headache. Headache, 34: 344–350.

Lerner, D., Adler, D., Chang, H., et al. (2004) Unemployment, job retention and productivity loss among employees with depression. Psychiatr. Serv., 55: 1371–1378.

Loomis, R. (2005) Relation of psychosocioeconomic variables and elapsed time out of work to intent to return to work among chronic pain patients. Dissertation Abstracts International. Section B: The Sciences and Engineering, 65(10B): 5411.

Naidoo, P. and Pillay, Y. (1994) Correlations among general stress, family environment, psychological distress, and pain experience. Percept. Mot. Skills, 78: 1291–1296.

Nicassio, P. and Radojevic, V. (1993) Models of family functioning and their contribution to patient's outcome in chronic pain. Motiv. Emot., 17: 295–316.

Nicassio, P., Radojevic, V., Schofield-Smith, K., et al. (1995) The contribution of family cohesion and pain coping process to depression symptoms in fibromyalgia. Ann. Behav. Med., 17: 349–359.

Romano, J., Turner, J., and Jensen, M. (1997) The family environment in chronic pain patients: comparison to controls and relationships to patient functioning. J. Clin. Psychol. Health Settings, 4: 383–395.

Roy, R. (2001) Social Relations and Chronic Pain. New York, Kluwer/Plenum.

Roy, R. (2006) Chronic Pain and Family: A Clinical Perspective. New York, Springer.

Roy, R. (2007) Social dislocation and the chronic pain patient. In: Bond, M. (Ed.) Encyclopedia of Pain. Heidelberg, Germany, Springer.

Roy, R. and Thomas, M. (1989) Nature of marital relations among chronic pain patients. Contemp. Fam. Ther., 11: 277–284.

Smith, R. (1998) Impact of migraine on the family. Headache, 38: 424–426.

Stang, P., Von Korff, M., and Galer, B. (1998) Reduced labor force participation among primary care patients with headaches. J. Gen. Intern. Med., 13: 296–302.

Thomas, M. and Roy, R. (1999) The Changing Nature of Pain over the Life-Span. New York, Plenum.

Turner, J. and Turner, R. (2004) Physical disability, unemployment and mental health. Rehabil. Psychol., 49: 241–249.

Warwick, R., Joseph, S., Cordle, C., and Ashworth, P. (2004) Social support for women with chronic pelvic pain: what is helpful for whom? Psychol. Health, 19: 117–134.

Watson, P., Booker, C., Moores, L., et al. (2004) Returning the chronically unemployed with low back pain to employment. Eur. J. Pain, 8: 359–369.

Chapter 3
Family Therapy and Couple Therapy

Family Therapy

Since we conducted a major review of the efficacy of family therapy more than a decade ago and concluded that family therapy was indeed effective with selected populations, but in the absence of evidence for its efficacy with the medically ill population in general and the chronic pain population in particular, a great deal of new information has emerged (Roy and Frankel, 1995). Before we consider the usefulness of family therapy for patients with chronic pain, we report on, first, reviews of family therapy effectiveness over the past ten years and, second, reviews that have used meta-analyses to ascertain the effectiveness of family therapy in general.

Disruption in family function is not an uncommon occurrence in families with a chronic pain sufferer in their midst. As was noted in the preceding chapter, the consequences can be far reaching. Of course, not all such families are equally affected. Some adapt very well to their altered circumstances. However, patients who are more disabled, such as many of those we tend to see in a pain clinic setting, do not. First, we present two cases to determine the efficacy of family therapy, with one case being more successful than the other; second, we review the literature to ascertain the efficacy of family therapy in general terms; and third, the efficacy with the medically ill populations. Does the evidence justify family therapy with the chronic pain population?

Case Illustrations

Before presenting the cases, a few general observations are in order. In a pain clinic setting, the families are seen usually at the request of the therapists. Motivation of patients/families to engage in therapy varies, and it is not unusual for one partner to be more invested than the other. Rate of attrition seems to be high, although there is no data to support this observation. It is a rare event when a patient actually asks for a family session. The purpose of therapy is not usually directly related to the goal of amelioration of pain. Rather, the objective is to ease the tension in the family system,

R. Roy, *Psychosocial Interventions for Chronic Pain*,
DOI: 10.1007/978-0-387-76296-8_3 © Springer Science+Business Media, LLC 2008

which is a consequence of changes brought about by illness in a family member, usually a parent and a partner. The inability of the patient to perform their normal roles, which in turn requires significant reorganization in the family structure, is often at the heart of family dissension and disagreement. Effective communication is a frequent casualty. Impact of illness on the children is often a major motivation to engage in family therapy.

The model of therapy used in treating the two families discussed here is systemic—a combination of Minuchin's structural model and the problem-centered approach developed by Epstein and colleagues, at the heart of which is the Mc-Master Model of Family Functioning (MMFF). We shall not describe the MMFF in detail here, and it has been extensively reported elsewhere by this author in the assessment of chronic pain families (Roy, 1989, 2006). Suffice it to say that MMFF measures family functioning along the dimensions of problem-solving, communication, role performance, affective involvement, affective responsiveness, and behavior control.

A Case of Successful Outcome?

Joan, a professional woman in her early forties, was referred to a pain clinic by her neurologist, who stated that the patient had other "unresolved" issues in her life which were having an impact on her headache. Joan had a very long history of migraine-type headache, which had worsened. She was asked to bring her husband for the initial interview, but she came alone. She was very well dressed and had a friendly demeanor. She did not give any outward evidence of pain, and in fact, that day she was pain-free.

Joan was extraordinarily articulate. She informed the therapist that she was having a few arguments with her husband because of the fact that she felt deeply indebted to him for accepting her pain and periodic disability and because she rarely offered any opinion on decisions that had to be made. In addition, her 8-year-old daughter frequently expressed concern about her headaches and tended to cling to her, and this was worrying. Her 6-year-old daughter seemed unaffected. Her husband played a major role in raising the children, which was another source of guilt for our patient. The frequency of her headaches had increased, and she was told by her neurologist that stressors in her life were probably contributing to her pain. She never complained of pain to her family, and when the pain was truly severe she would retreat to bed. She wondered if the clinic could be of any help to her. Our suggestion to involve her family in therapy was not well received. She claimed that it would be a further burden on her husband. In any event, she was the one who had the problems, not her husband. It took some persuasion to make her agree to be seen jointly with her husband, and later in therapy her older daughter was also brought in.

On the second visit, she was accompanied by her husband George. He was also a professional and between the two of them they had a substantial income. It did not take him long to state his central concern about their relationship: Joan was very reluctant to engage in any discussion that required decision making—whether it meant buying a new car or choice of a school for their daughters. At the end he had to decide alone, and he was becoming a little resentful. Of course, he never knew when she was in the throes of her headache unless she was in bed. Perhaps, he felt,he took on too much responsibility to protect her and now she was disengaged. Joan more or less agreed with George except his claim that she was disengaged.

On the basis of the MMFF, a somewhat different picture emerged. These were responsible parents who believed in sharing equally their responsibilities, always consulting each other on money matters, and sharing household chores. However, their role performance was modestly compromised owing to Joan's periodic headaches, during which phase she was quite incapacitated. George had to pitch in, but he was beginning to be angry about the unpredictability of these events, especially as Joan was less than verbal about her pain and George usually had to guess that she had headaches except when her pain was severe and she was in bed. This also interfered to a certain extent with their social engagements, of which they had many.

They both acknowledged that they had experienced some problems around communication. Joan felt deeply obligated to George and felt that she had no right to be critical of him. George was very sympathetic of Joan's problems, but he did wish she would be more forthcoming with her pain. He had learned to hold his tongue, but sometimes he felt very frustrated.

They enjoyed their sexual relations, which was somewhat unpredictable owing to Joan's headaches. They did try to involve each other in making major decisions, although George felt that Joan depended too much on him. They were equally involved in the lives of their young children and both acknowledged each other as a very caring parent. They had concerns about their 8-year-old, who was very worried about her mother and tended to cling to her.

In broad terms, this was a functioning family where chronic pain in a partner and parent created some very predictable problems. However, their perception of the problems was quite different.

The dynamics of their problem is all too familiar to anyone working with chronic pain families. The well-partner (George) wants to protect the sick-partner (Joan) from day-to-day trials and tribulations. The sick-partner feels obligated (and in Joan's case, guilt) and lives with the dual feelings of obligation and even gratefulness and of the sense of losing the right to say anything at all. Over time, George finds himself making all kinds of decisions without the benefit of Joan's input and becomes resentful. Joan continues to act on her guilt and obligation and behaves as some one without any say. Not a very satisfactory situation. One child, in the meantime, shows signs of anxiety over mother's condition and tends to regress. The reality, however, was that although they harbored some of the feelings they shared with the therapist, their behavior suggested a far less serious situation.

The actual therapy in this case was quite simple. Joan did not have a debilitating disease. For the most part, she lived a relatively normal life. She did not have to depend on George to the extent that she had learned to be or she thought she was (with George's well-meaning collusion), and she could indeed regain some of her influence in family matters. In fact, she had retained much of that influence. George was all for it, but he also needed to know when she was in pain. He behaved as though her pain was continuous. His task was not to view Joan as disabled, but rather as a person who functioned at a very high level much of the time.

They had four sessions over a period of just more than 2 months, and one of the sessions included their older daughter. This daughter received a great deal of reassurance from both parents, reinforced by the therapist, that her mother's problem was not serious and that she suffered from a common headache problem which sometimes got bad. Assumption of conjugal and parental roles on the part of Joan, both of which had been somewhat compromised in Joan's mind, and George's shift in attitude and behavior toward his wife's level of disability contributed to a significant degree to the amelioration of their conflict

Rationale for family therapy was self-evident in this case. Sporadic pain in one partner created a cycle of behaviors that was beginning to have an effect on the couple's relationship. Nevertheless, their functioning was virtually at the healthy end of the continuum. Outcome could be construed as positive. Six-month follow-up showed that they were maintaining their improvements. Their daughter was no longer anxious. George had stopped viewing his wife as disabled and Joan, in her turn, was more verbal about her pain, and her sense of guilt was significantly ameliorated. They were discharged from the clinic and Joan was referred back to her neurologist. Finally, it must be noted that this was mainly a well-functioning family that required some minimal adjustments. The positive outcome was not a surprise. Our next case tells a different story.

A Family That Wouldn't Engage

Sam, in his mid-forties, was referred to our pain clinic for persistent pain in his arm and neck, the origin of which was uncertain. Comprehensive investigation to detect the cause of his pain and spasm had proven negative. He was on a heavy dose of narcotic analgesics, which kept him functioning. He was still very functional and worked in his own business for ten or more hours a day. He had to be on his feet much of that time.

Sam was married with two children. His wife Pat was a healthcare professional and also worked full-time. He was very truculent in the beginning stages of therapy, and it was a while before he began to express conflicts within his family. He had two major issues. The first was his wife's reluctance to accept his pain problem and her serious objection to him ingesting "a vast quantity of poison" to control his pain. The second was his ongoing battle with his daughter, whom he regarded as disrespectful and who was always defended by her mother. It was proposed that the whole family should be seen, to which he agreed. However, he could not speak for Pat.

The first family session was quite remarkable for a number of reasons. Despite our request to bring the children, only Sam and his wife Pat showed up. Pat was very smartly dressed and had overtly easy manners. Her exterior calm was deceptive as within a minute or two into the session, she broke down. Sam showed no inclination to reach out and comfort her, but maintained his cool distance. During the entire session, they failed to have any eye contact.

Nevertheless, some salient points emerged. Sam had become impossible to live with. He was angry all the time and the children were fearful of their father. No, he was never physically violent, but he could be very loud. She was forced into siding with the daughter in particular, because he was super critical of her. He got along much better with his son. Sam sat impassively. Finally, he demanded that Pat reveal to the therapist reason for his anger, and he added that she had alienated him from the children. Sam spent his evenings by himself in the basement and he was like a lodger in his own house. He barely participated in the lives of his children and the entire responsibility fell on the shoulders of Pat. There ensued a great deal of mutual recrimination, at the heart of which was his over-reliance on very powerful narcotic analgesics and his anger. On his part, he tried to defend himself and then gave up and retreated into silence. This was how the first session ended and they agreed that on their next visit they would bring their daughter. They never returned as a family. Sam remained in psychotherapy for some length of time.

On the MMFF, this family seemed to be at the least-effective end virtually on all the dimensions. From their problem-solving ability to their ability to be consistent in their rules for children were all to one extent or another compromised. Communication was minimal between the two partners. Sam was disengaged from the family affairs to the point that he was very much like a lodger in his own home. He did have a close relationship with his son. He explained that his son was the main reason why he had not separated. His wife had threatened separation on many occasions, but had not acted on her threats. This family's problems pre-dated the onset of Sam's health problems and his medical condition(s) only exacerbated an already compromised situation.

Failure of family therapy in a case where therapy was clearly indicated could be attributed to a number of factors, the principal one being the motivation of the family members. This is a serious issue in a secondary setting such as a pain clinic. Patients do not normally seek family therapy, and it often takes some persuasion to get families to participate in this activity. Problems are twofold: first, sometimes patients are unwilling to involve their partners and children in therapy, and second, many families do not remain engaged after their initial involvement. Unfortunately, at the time of writing, there is no data available to show the rate of attrition of families in a pain clinic setting. Many patients and their partners express a common sentiment that their purpose of being in a pain clinic is to have their pain "fixed." Once that goal is achieved, all other problems would disappear.

Sam outwardly gave the impression of being willing to engage, but he showed no further inclination to do so. His attitude was that his wife in particular was against him because she showed a total lack of understanding of his pain condition and treated him like a drug addict. Pat, when reached by phone, was equally reluctant to return for therapy. Her view was uncomplicated. His pain had no physical basis and he should not be on all that medication. It was the medication that had changed her husband and turned him into a hostile and angry man and no amount of therapy was going to change that. Their respective attitudes suggested some long-standing conflicts in this marriage. Therapy in this case ended almost before it began. Nevertheless, this intervention has to be viewed as a failure.

The two cases we described above fall into the category of medical family therapy. We shall now review the literature on the outcome of medical family therapy, but in the context of the efficacy of family therapy in general.

Family Therapy and Outcome

Reviews on the outcome of family therapy tend to be quite positive. Carr (2000), for instance, in his presentation of evidence for the efficacy of family therapy, pronounced that this form of psychotherapy had indeed come of age, and was effective in dealing with a whole range of problems and issues, including chronic pain.

Carr (2000) cast a rather wide net that covered many divergent types of intervention that may or may not include more than one member of the family. He investigated eight areas, namely, marital problems, relationship problems, psychosexual problems, anxiety disorders, mood disorders, alcohol abuse, chronic pain management, and family management of neurologically impaired adults. However, he pointed out that six of the eight problems listed above were framed in individualistic rather than systemic terms. This was in contrast to the review of Roy and Frankel (1995), which focused on systemic family therapy and arrived at a much less optimistic conclusion than Carr's. In their attempt to answer the question "How good is family therapy?" they concluded that family therapy had yet to make a strong and persuasive case for its effectiveness based on hard data. Controlled studies in this domain were found to be few and far between. However, the literature on the merit of family therapy for health problems includes studies on stroke (Clark et al., 2003), cancer (Keller and Jost, 2003; Sellers, 2000), diabetes (Hagglund et al., 1996; Satin, 1989), and depression (Chase and Holmes, 1990; Clarkin et al., 1990; Lebow and Gurman, 1995; Stevenson, 1993; Waring et al., 1995).

However, based on what he derived from research evidence, Carr was very convincing about the effectiveness of family therapy. In the context of different reviewers using different definitions of what may or may not be family therapy, Rivett and Street (2003) noted that such definitional variations resulted in different conclusions. That was how they accounted for Carr's optimistic assessment as opposed to Roy and Frankel's qualified perspective. The review that follows adheres in broad terms to the systemic family therapy literature, and attempts to assess the progress made over the past 10 years in family therapy outcome research.

A more recent review (Clarkin et al., 2003) reached conclusions similar to Carr's (2000). These authors also adopted a very broad definition of family therapy which ranged from working with the spouse alone to psychoeducational programs to family groups. Under the heading of "review of well-designed studies," they listed difficulties in the parent–child relationship, specific problems related to children, non-specific parent–adolescent conflicts, adolescent behavior problems and delinquency, substance abuse, eating disorders, schizophrenia, and affective disorders. They concluded that the methodology in family therapy research was improving. However, in areas such as eating disorders, substance abuse, and affective disorders, a more refined research methodology was called for. A vast majority of the studies reported in their review used cognitive behavioral techniques, and more importantly, other techniques were more the exceptions.

Only a handful of studies used systemic approaches. They related to a comparison of parent training and multisystemic therapy (MST) for child abuse and neglect (Brunk et al., 1987), treatment of anorexia nervosa (Crisp et al., 1991), family therapy for disturbed children (Garrigan and Bambrick, 1977), family therapy with adolescents (Guldner, 1990), drug abuse (Henggeler, 1993), and family therapy in an inpatient setting (Ro-Trock et al., 1977). Three studies compared structural/systemic therapy with another competing strategy (Barkley et al., 1992; Stanton et al., 1982; Szykula et al., 1987). One point of note was that the reports showed that family therapy using cognitive behavioral techniques was most commonly subjected to the rigor of randomized trials. The overall tone of the reviews was optimistic.

Evidence-based reports on the efficacy of family therapy with children with attention deficit disorder (Bjornstad and Montgomery, 2006), with youth aged 10–17 having social and emotional problems (Littell et al., 2006), and with children with asthma (Yorke and Shuldham, 2006) have been published as Cochrane Reviews. We report briefly on these findings. Two studies related to the treatment of attention deficit disorder that met the Cochrane Review treatment criteria, which are very stringent and include only RCTs, have been reviewed. Data extracted from both studies indicated that no difference could be detected between the efficacy of behavioral family therapy and that of the usual treatment in the community.

Another review examined the efficacy of family therapy for social, emotional, and behavioral problems in youth aged 10–17 and reached the following conclusion (Littell et al., 2006). Results of eight RCTs conducted across a number of countries showed that any firm conclusion about the effectiveness of multisystemic family therapy would be premature. Results were inconsistent across the studies and varied in quality. There was no information about the effects of MST compared to no treatment. MST was found not to produce any negative effects.

The focus of the third review was to assess the efficacy of systemic family therapy for the treatment of chronic asthma, and it included two randomized trials with a total of 55 children (Yorke and Shuldham, 2006). The findings could not be combined because of the different outcome measures adopted by the studies. The authors concluded that family therapy may be a useful adjunct to medication for children with asthma. However, the low sample sizes in the two studies and lack of standardized outcome measures were deemed to be limiting factors.

These three reviews, with stringent criteria for inclusion and all of them with children, produced only nominal evidence for the efficacy of family therapy. In fact, family therapy in conjunction with medication proved efficacious only with pediatric asthma. In short, effectiveness of family therapy remains questionable. It is worth reiterating that Cochrane Reviews demand the highest standard of proof, that is, RCTs, to demonstrate efficacy of treatment. We shall revisit the question of standard of proof throughout this volume. Based on the above reports, a rather pessimistic view could be that not much has changed over the years in the way of establishing new and convincing evidence for the efficacy of family therapy with children.

Campbell and Patterson (1995) produced a lengthy report on the effectiveness of family interventions in the treatment of physical illness. This is what they wrote about the state of family therapy with children: "Although the results of these studies (five studies on family therapy), are promising, confidence in the efficacy and effectiveness of family therapy in treating children's physical illness is still limited because of inadequate study designs: no control group, very small sample sizes, no standardized measure of impact, and/or lack of control of other confounding variables" (pp. 549, 554). A less optimistic view would be that the Cochrane group, which requires very rigorous research design, managed to conduct three reviews on the merit of family therapy with the pediatric population.

In their review of family therapy with the adult medically ill population, Campbell and Patterson (1995) reached similarly pessimistic conclusions. Their overall assessment was that, at the time of writing, there was a complete absence of any kind of controlled trials of family therapy for chronic adult physical illnesses. They reviewed the pertinent literature on cardiovascular disease, neurological disorders, and obesity. Despite lack of evidence, they concluded that research supported the increasingly important role of medical family therapy. Campbell (2002) more recently observed that although there exists a large body of research on the impact of marriage on chronic illness and overall health, and on overall family functioning , there are very few reports on family therapy and no randomized control trials exist for family therapy with adult physical illness.

Moreover, review of more recent literature on medical family therapy tends to confirm the observations of Campbell and Patterson (1995) made over a decade ago. In an otherwise excellent paper on medical family therapy, Sholevar and Sahar (2003) failed to provide any tangible evidence for the efficacy of family therapy with the medically ill populations. In fact, they drew on rather dated literature (on some occasions) to find justification for family therapy. An illustration of that is their description of the "psychosomatic" model, along with structural family therapy which was developed by Minuchin (1974). They provided one more reference that dated back to 1974. The fact is that this model has not received any significant empirical support; however, it is noteworthy structural therapy has been demonstrated to be somewhat effective with conditions such as pediatric asthma and anorexia nervosa.

Roy and Frankel (1995), writing on family therapy and pediatric asthma, noted that three controlled family therapy outcome studies, taken together, began to make a case for the efficacy of family therapy (Backman et al., 1981; Gustafsson et al., 1986; Lask and Matthew, 1979). Furthermore, they reported that the findings of the family-oriented studies were also positive. As was noted earlier, even with the stringent criteria of Cochrane Reviews, family therapy for pediatric asthma as an adjunct is meritorious.

Summary

All the major reviews about the current health of family therapy generally arrive at a rather optimistic conclusion. On the other hand, family therapy with medically ill adults awaits empirical validation. Yet, an argument can be made that medical family therapy shares much with family therapy with families facing interpersonal difficulties. Consensus is emerging from among a divergent set of reviews using rather disparate definitions of family therapy and equally disparate measures of the efficacy of family therapy. If we return to our case illustrations at the very beginning of this chapter, we can clearly see that the success of the family therapy with the first case could be attributed to the obvious interpersonal difficulties this family encountered owing to chronic pain. Indeed, other factors such as motivation and premorbid functioning also contributed to their success. The point is that the cause of family dissension may vary, but the effectiveness of family therapy in repairing faulty or strained relationship has more general application.

Meta-Analysis

We now turn our attention to reports that used meta-analysis to assess family therapy outcome. Meta-analysis involves the use of quantitative techniques to summarize the results of scientific studies on the same question. An important innovation in meta-analysis was the use of an effect size as a common metric over different studies to measure how large is the effect of a treatment (Shadish and Baldwin, 2003).

There are only very few reports on the meta-analysis of the effectiveness of family therapy. A PsycINFO search using the keywords "family therapy and meta-analyses" produced only eight results. Overall, the results of these reports are encouraging. Sack and Thomasius (2002) concluded on the basis their meta-analysis that family therapy was an appropriate treatment for adolescent drug abuse and drug dependency. In meta-analysis, family therapy revealed medium-sized effects and superior outcome, in treatment of both children and adolescents.

Shadish and Baldwin (2003) conducted one of the most comprehensive reviews of meta-analysis of marital and family therapy (MFT) literature. We report their findings in some detail. They summarized the overall results of 20 meta-analyses that were done on the effects of both therapy and enrichment interventions with couples and families. In their review of MFT versus controls, they concluded that MFT interventions were effective. In direct comparisons between different kinds of MFTs, they reported on four meta-analyses, and found that no significant differences existed between various models of MFT.

In terms of clinical significance of MFT, their conclusion was that marriage and family therapies produced clinically significant improvements in distressed clients, with success rates of between 40% and 50%. Their overall conclusion on the efficacy of MFT was that, first, MFTs were clearly efficacious compared to no treatment. Second, those interventions were at least as effective as other types of interventions such individual psychotherapy, and perhaps more effective in at least some cases. Third, there was little evidence for differential efficacy among the various approaches to marriage and family interventions, especially if mediating and moderating variables were controlled. Finally, and perhaps most importantly, evidence that MFT interventions were effective in clinically representative conditions remained sparse, although there were a few exceptions to that. They ended their

comprehensive review on an optimistic note. They stated that "the work we reviewed
... shows that marriage and family therapy is now an empirically supported therapy
in the plain English sense of the phrase—both in general and for a variety of specific
problems." The MFT interventions covered in this report were with many different
populations, the exception being the medically or the physically ill or disabled. The
question, however, remains as to whether, given the overall success of MFT, there
is reason to be optimistic about its benefits for the medically ill population. In fact,
the review that we would discuss next has considerable relevance to the physically
ill and relatives' burden of care is a relatively well-researched topic.

Cuijpers (1999) conducted a meta-analysis of the effects of family interventions
on relatives' burden of caring for patients with schizophrenia. Sixteen studies were
included in this analysis. In 14 of these studies, an experimental condition was
compared to a control group or two interventions were compared to each other.
Somewhat disparate outcome measures were used by the studies and the sample
sizes tended to be small. The elements of burden that were investigated were very
heterogeneous. Family interventions ranged from a single educational session to
intensive family therapy. A point of note is that family functioning, which was described variously as family conflict, family disruption, interference with family life,
family satisfaction, and family distress, was the focal point of eight studies. In other
words, these studies employed a systemic approach to treat these families. This is an
important point as families having a member with chronic pain generally encounter
a similar set of problems, and systems-based family therapy in those circumstances
could be seen as the therapy of choice.

Despite these limitations, Cuijpers (1999) concluded that family interventions
with relatives of psychiatric patients could significantly reduce their burden in caring
for the patients. Because of family interventions, improvement in the family's psychological distress, relationship between patient and relative, and in overall family
functioning was found. Another finding of some importance, in this day and age of
brief therapy, was that interventions with 12 sessions or more were more effective
than shorter interventions.

Summary

What conclusions can be drawn from the meta-analysis literature on the efficacy of
family therapy? Broadly, family therapy is effective in many different settings and
in dealing with an assortment of family difficulties. The conclusion of both Shadish
and Baldwin (2003) and Cuijpers (1999) points in the direction that systems-based
family therapy has indeed received substantial empirical validation to justify the use
of family therapy in addressing interpersonal and relationship problems under many
conditions. It is worth reiterating that Cuijpers' findings are of special relevance to
chronic pain patients as many families facing this problem experience a great deal
of stress owing to shift in responsibilities from the sick partner to the well partner.
Proof of this observation is to be found in the fact that spouses (wives) of chronic
pain sufferers are vulnerable to depression, one of the causes of which is the added
burden (Roy, 2006).

Family Therapy and Chronic Pain

One inescapable conclusion, on the basis of the major reviews presented here, was that the efficacy determined primarily based on RCTs of family therapy for adult physical illness is yet to emerge. With that in mind, we turn our attention to family therapy for chronic pain management and attempt to simply ascertain, in the first place, what and how much has been written on this topic and second, evaluate their merit for effectiveness.

A PsycINFO search from 1974 to the present (March 2006) using the keywords "chronic pain and family therapy" yielded 61 results. Preponderance of clinical papers is only eclipsed by the absence of empirically validated reports on the effectiveness of family therapy. Besides, several articles produced by this search had no relevance to the topic at hand. One qualitative study, however, reported on the benefits of family discussion groups (FDG), which involved 19 chronic pain patients, 41 family members, 8 therapists, and 17 observers (Lemmens et al., 2003). These subjects were divided into four FDGs. Every FDG cycle consisted of five sessions and lasted about 90 minutes each. This was not strictly an outcome study, but was designed to determine the extent to which therapists and patients/families valued various elements of their group therapy experience. Events helpful for the individual, the family, and the group were explored after each session with evaluation questionnaires. Evaluation showed that the therapeutic team and the families experienced many helpful events during the FDG sessions.

The therapeutic team regarded the relational climate and the specific interventions as their focus. Families, on the other hand, found the process aspect of the group intervention as particularly useful. The authors observed that "The chronic pain patients and their family members benefit mostly from becoming conscious of/gaining insight into the family, and to a lesser extent in the illness and oneself. Although no specific information or education about family or illness issues were given by therapists, the variety of different and similar stories between the group members . . . in the FDG are likely to have stimulated different cognitive processes, which helped patients and families who were often only focused directly on the pain problems and involved in rigid interactions, to broaden their viewpoints." That the group experience was beneficial for the patients and their families was beyond question.

Roy (1989, 2001, 2006) has reported extensively on the use of Problem-Centered Systemic Family Therapy (PCSFT), at the core of which is the MMFF, in treating families with chronic pain patients. He has pointed out the therapy's strengths and weaknesses and has suggested modification of the model under certain conditions. Roy (1989) described family functioning on the basis of MMFF of 32 patients (20 with headache and 12 with chronic back pain) and their families. Family therapy based on PCSFT was found useful by 16 families in the headache group and only four in the back pain group. This study was clinical in nature, but incorporated some of the elements of a qualitative study. Can it be argued that this particular body of literature provides some evidence to justify family therapy with families with chronic pain patients?

Roy's (2006) recent review noted that no controlled studies existed on family therapy and chronic pain. In fact, the picture is bleak as research into the family issues of chronic pain sufferers has come to a virtual stop (2006). Yet, the clinical literature can only be described as rich. Is that body of literature of any value for justification of family therapy with this population? The fact that chronic pain is capable of disrupting family function is not debatable. Also, the fact that family members and the patient experience various degrees of distress is beyond question. A strict view would be to acknowledge that family therapy for chronic pain must await clinical trials analogous to drug trials. This means, until family therapy is proven to be effective, this treatment should not be offered. That is neither tenable nor practical.

The necessity of intervention in the case of Joan and her young family, discussed at the beginning of this chapter, was almost self-evident. The goal was clear. Unless the problems of Joan and her husband George were addressed, there was a real chance that they would get entrenched in them and their relationship would take a downward slide. Their child's anxiety about her mother's health also had to be tackled. Under these circumstances, what part should the absence of empirical support play in the decision to offer family therapy? A related question is the cumulative value of clinical evidence and qualitative information in the decision-making process to offer family therapy. Can some generalizable conclusions be drawn from this case?

First and foremost, a family harboring a chronically sick individual encounters problems that are well documented in the literature. Situations like the above case demand intervention. In such a situation, the high bar of proven therapy based on RCTs is not sustainable. Less formidable evidence has to be sought. We have argued that extrapolation from the general effectiveness of family therapy in redressing faulty family relationship must be imported into treating families with chronic pain patients. Clinical literature in support of this therapy cannot and should not be discounted. Perhaps it is worthy of reiteration that family therapy with this population is not designed to ameliorate or eliminate pain, but rather the goal is to enable the families to deal more effectively with changing circumstances. Hence, a point made earlier, namely that family therapy has been shown to be effective in treating relationship problems, is worth recalling. Further weight is added to this argument by the conclusions of Cuijpers (1999).

Let us return to our second case where a family (Sam and Pat) failed to engage, and analyze what was at stake for this family. This was indeed a family in a high level of distress. Prima facie, this family's lack of motivation may be viewed as the sole reason for their unwillingness. Or, one party or the other had already decided that their problems were beyond repair. Or, they had arrived at a point where they were accepting of their situation and indeed found a way of living with each other. Perhaps, it was a combination of all these factors. In fact Sam on one occasion informed his therapist that he was unwilling to leave this marriage as long as the children were young.

Yet, even from a pain management point of view, the family situation was wanting. Pat's unwillingness to accept Sam's legitimate treatment was certainly adding to the distress level of the patient. That family therapy in this case was called for would be hard to ignore. This case was not in the category of treatment failure, but in that of failure to engage. Research, as well as clinical literature in family therapy, is somewhat silent on treatment failures or clinicians' inability to engage some families.

Summary

First and foremost, medical family therapy is yet to come of age. Second, the necessity of family therapy with chronic pain patients and their families is beyond question. There are three kinds of evidence that may be considered as basis for family therapy with this population:

1. Clinical and limited research literature that exists on medical family therapy, despite some serious methodological gaps, seems promising;
2. Extrapolation from MFT literature shows both MFT's effectiveness in addressing interpersonal issues and that it holds considerable promise. Interpersonal difficulties are commonly reported by our patients and have received some empirical validation.
3. Evidence points out that the question of efficacy should be transcended as the need for family intervention, as demonstrated even by our two cases, remains paramount. A critical point made by Shadish and Baldwin (2003) was that family therapy was more effective than no treatment. For the moment, until further research, we have to assume that this is indeed so. Nevertheless, practitioners need a heightened level of awareness that family therapy with chronic pain patients remains somewhat of an uncharted territory. Their patients are also entitled to this information.

Couple Therapy

We begin our discussion about couple therapy with two case illustrations. The first case involves a couple in their sixties and the second, a couple in their twenties. Pain was implicated in both cases, but in vastly different ways. Our focus, however, remains on how the relationships were directly or not so directly influenced by the fact of one partner having a chronic pain problem.

Case Illustrations

Margaret, aged 67, was referred to our clinic following a rather dramatic deterioration in her headache and back pain. Neurological and orthopedic investigations to detect the cause were negative. She had a lifelong history of headaches, which had not presented a serious challenge to her well-being. Her back pain was also of some 25 years' duration. Despite her prolonged history of pain, she had led a full life.

She had hardly ever sought medical help with her pain. However, on this occasion, she consulted her family physician and she was prescribed powerful analgesics and antidepressants, but without any positive outcome.

Margaret along with her husband Jo was seen for routine psychosocial investigation. They had a traditional marriage in that Jo was the main breadwinner and Margaret, a homemaker. Jo was a successful businessman and for much of his working life had traveled round the world, spending little time at home. Margaret raised five children "almost single-handed," she claimed. She described her husband as somewhat peripheral to the family system, though in recent years he had grown closer to the children. He angrily rejected her description of his peripheral role. He held a very responsible position which had kept him away from his family, but he tried very hard to be around as much as he could. He portrayed his wife as a perfectionist, overbearing, and always expecting too much from him. Despite these chronic conflicts, all five children were pursuing successful careers in various professions. They acknowledged that since Jo's retirement, their relationship had deteriorated rather sharply. This was the first indication of a major, though not unexpected, life event they had recently experienced.

Since his retirement, Jo had intruded into her daily life in a wholly unacceptable way. He showed very little regard for her daily routine, and sat reading the newspaper in the kitchen for hours on end. He refused to shave unless he had to, and worst of all wore the same underclothes for 2 or 3 days in a row. Then there was a dramatic development. He claimed serious hearing loss.

Margaret would be blasting away at him about this and that, and he would sit without as much as moving a muscle. This drove Margaret to distraction. He was examined by the family physician, who could not find any hearing abnormality. Margaret's headaches took a turn for the worse, which seriously affected her day-to-day life. On some days she could not even get out of bed. On these occasions, Jo would be a changed man, being overly solicitous and "unendingly" fussing over his wife. As soon as her headaches improved, he would return to his "obnoxious self."

The major life event for Margaret and Jo was indeed Jo's retirement. This is not necessarily undesirable and most certainly is predictable. In that sense, this event did not have to be perceived as negative. Jo's attitude toward retirement was mixed. He welcomed the absence of endless travel, which left him with ample time to "please himself." He missed his lifelong friends in the business world, but he had joined a golf club to compensate for that. Margaret's response was almost entirely negative. This only worsened with each passing day. She saw him as lazy, uncooperative, and generally a nuisance.

Margaret was reluctant to invite her friends home to save herself the "embarrassment" of exposing her unkempt husband, and her worsening pain prevented her from remaining engaged in the community. Jo, as stated, missed his friends from work, but this did not leave a very serious gap in his life. He was busy planning for his retired existence.

In terms of family relationship, the role of retirement and Margaret's pain problems were quite revealing. From the view of interpersonal relationships, the "message" value or the metaphorical aspect of Margaret's pain is instructive. At its simplest, the pain was a powerful message for expressing dissatisfaction with her life situation precipitated by her husband's retirement. At a more complex level, pain helped to level "hierarchical incongruity." This concept is predicated on the assumption that although a symptomatic partner in a marriage assumes a dependent position, symptoms also have the capacity to empower that person, which, in turn, rectifies the power imbalance in marriage (Madanes, 1981).

In short, pain enables the person in the lower position to gain the upper hand. Jo, having lost his power and authority in the business world, reacted by becoming a "slob". He virtually destroyed Margaret's assumptive world, and the control she had exercised over this world all her married life. His desire to basically ignore her world was challenged only when Margaret's pain reached a high level of disability. In that situation, Margaret regained some of her authority by forcing him into an unfamiliar nurturing role, and on these occasions Margaret was listened to literally and figuratively. Margaret regained some of her power by becoming symptomatic. Here, it must be emphasized that the mechanism involved in Margaret's increasing pain is far from simple. It is almost always unconscious, and frequently, psychophysiological processes, such as increased stress contributing to more muscle tension and more pain, may be involved.

Marital therapy was implemented. This therapy, based on PCSFT, which is behavior oriented, worked well for this couple. They had to develop some new rules and discover new ways of relating to one another. In the course of this therapy, two measurable improvements occurred. Margaret's headaches became less intense and less frequent and Jo seemed to make a remarkable recovery from his "deafness." Following the completion of this therapy and a 6 month follow-up, Margaret was discharged from the clinic.

Our second case involves two young people. June, in her late twenties, was referred to the pain clinic by her neurosurgeon for pain management related to post-operative pain following several resections for low-grade glioma in the thalamic region. She complained of pain in the left side of the body, which she described as "shooting", and lacerating pain that could be tingling, hurting, and tender.

June and her husband Robert were seen for routine psychosocial evaluation, and very soon in the session, marital discord between the two of them surfaced. The core of the complaint was that June, who despite her pain worked full-time, was "lazy" around the house. June defended herself vigorously by pointing out that she was working full-time and was bringing home more money. Admittedly, she missed work owing to pain three or four times a month. She had very understanding employers and they were willing to make concessions because of her health problems. Robert was working part-time and studying as well. He was extremely busy and countered by saying that any help around the house would be deeply appreciated. Robert remained tearful throughout the session. He was discouraged and demoralized. Any kind of social life for them was absent and between the two of them they had very little social support. It became apparent that Robert was struggling with coming to terms with the fact that so soon in their marriage he had a sick partner, and he was simply unwilling to accept that fact. He had made very little effort to educate himself about June's complex medical condition and seemed mired in his own disappointment. They were offered conjoint therapy and they agreed.

Robert knew even before his marriage that June had significant health problems, but was optimistic that her health would improve. He still could not figure out how June was able to work full-time but was totally dependent on him for everything else. June, on the other hand, was becoming increasingly despondent. Their life was almost totally devoid of any enjoyment. Sex was sporadic.

Clinical focus shifted somewhat from the marital issues to June's psychiatric state, although the two were inextricably intertwined. Very little progress was witnessed from session to session. They returned more or less with the same issues. So far they have been seen for four sessions, which have not borne any significant results. In fact, Robert's ongoing complaints and criticism have had a direct impact on June's emotional state. In the last little while, she had entertained suicidal ideas. She complained of low mood and not feeling well. She was referred back to her family physician for an evaluation of her mood and need for medication. Conjoint therapy remains in a state of suspension as they failed to turn up for their last appointment.

There can be little argument that Robert seemed unprepared to cope with the ups and downs of June's medical condition. He was unable to fully accept that he had married an unwell individual and their marital relations would not resemble a couple of their age. He was disappointed. June, on her part, experienced heightened guilt emanating from Robert's criticisms and became increasingly depressed. The clinic continues to hope that they will return for therapy. At this point we turn our attention to the literature on couple therapy to establish the overall efficacy of couple therapy in general and for chronic pain disorders in particular.

Couple Therapy and Its Effectiveness

There appears to exist some level of consensus about the efficacy of couple therapy in addressing relationship issues. Johnson (2002), in a sweeping review of the marital problems and their treatment, and having pointed out many shortcomings in research, concluded that "The field of couples therapy appears to be in the process of integrating description, prediction, and explanation. Theory, practice, and systematic investigations are beginning to create a coherent whole" (pp. 182–183).

Johnson's assessment of the effectiveness of couple therapy for physical illness is encouraging. She cites a number of studies dealing with cancer and heart disease. Research shows that the quality of relationship between partners can have a significant impact on coping effectively with diverse conditions such as heart disease, breast cancer, and rheumatoid arthritis. We shall presently review some of that literature.

Johnson(2003), writing generally on the efficacy of couple therapy, noted that emotionally focused therapy (EFT) and behavioral marital therapy (BMT) are the only two interventions recognized by the American Psychological Association as effective. BMT demonstrated an effect size of 0.95. Johnson translated that to mean that the average person receiving BMT had higher scores on outcome measures than 83% of the untreated couples. EFT, which has been found to be effective with distressed couples, has also reported a high level of success. According to Johnson (2003), 70%–73% couples were found to be recovered from distress at follow-up after 10–12 sessions of EFT. Reports showed that this improvement was maintained over time.

Johnson (2003) ends her review on a positive note. While acknowledging that there is some distance yet to be traveled, couple therapy has gone through "a quantum leap in the quality and quantity of couples therapy research in the last decade. Methodologically sound research studies from different schools of couples therapy ... treatment implemented according to manuals, the use of implementation checks, control groups, follow-up results, and the reporting the rates of deterioration, are now becoming the norm" (p. 811).

More recent studies also confirm the general effectiveness of couple therapy (Baucom et al., 2003; Epstein, 2001; Leff et al., 2000; Olson, 2002; Snyder et al., 2006). We report briefly on a study by Leff and associates (2002) as this study met the criteria of RCTs. Leff et al. (2000) compared the relative efficacy and cost of couple therapy and antidepressant drugs for the treatment and maintenance of 77 people with depression who lived with a partner. An RCT of drug vs couple therapy was conducted. Of the participants, 56.8% dropped out from drug treatment and 15% from couple therapy. Improvement in depression was noted in both groups, but the couple therapy group showed a higher level of improvement on the Beck Depression Inventory, both at the end of treatment and at the 2-year follow-up. As for the cost, there were no appreciable differences between the two treatments. This study is of particular interest in relation to chronic pain patients as depression has been demonstrated to be consistently high in this population.

Summary

On the basis of this review, evidence points in the direction of considerable efficacy of couple therapy in lessening or even removing interpersonal problems. Although there is some debate about the orientation of therapy and what specific kind of problems may best respond to couple intervention, the findings are optimistic. In the section that follows, we review the efficacy of couple therapy with medical disorders including chronic pain problems.

Couple Therapy and Physical Illness (Chronic Pain)

Reports of couple therapy with the medically ill, including chronic pain sufferers and their partners, are few and far between. Most of the reports are of a clinical nature and even basic empirical studies, not to mention RCTs, are few and far between. However, we now report on a handful of studies that tend to suggest the merit of couple therapy with this population. Priebe and Sinning (2001) conducted an RCT in an investigation of the effects of a brief couple therapy for subjects and their partners in a cardiac rehabilitation program. A physician along with a psychologist conducted an intervention of 2–4 sessions with 19 patients with Stage II coronary diseases. Control group comprised of 21 patients who received standard care. Patients in the control group reported feeling better almost immediately after the intervention. Nine months later, the treatment group showed significantly more favorable changes. Authors concluded that a very short couple therapy intervention, which can be administered in routine care, could have positive effects in cardiac rehabilitation. They recommended large-scale replication of their study.

Webster (1992) described the efficacy of couple therapy in an uncontrolled study of 58 men with diabetes and accompanying sexual dysfunction. Apart from reporting clinical success of couple therapy, the necessity of undertaking routine couple intervention with diabetic patients and their partners was strongly urged.

Despite some limitations, research is broadly supportive of the operant behavioral paradigm on the spousal solicitous responses to pain behaviors. Although this approach has come under some criticism for its simplicity and lack of appreciation for all the complexities that surround this concept, from a treatment point of view this remains an important issue. Nevertheless, actual reports of treatment of this phenomena are very few.

Thieme and associates (2003) in a controlled study investigated 61 patients with fibromyalgia for the efficacy of operant pain treatment. The solicitous behavior of the spouse was assessed, and the overall objective of this project was to reduce patients' intake of pain medication, enhance physical activity, reduce pain's interference with family life, and train the family to avoid assertive pain-incompatible behavior. Results showed a marked reduction in the spouses' solicitous behaviors, and improvements were noted on all the other measures. Point of note, however, is that spousal involvement in this project was indirect as patients were given homework to facilitate an increase in activities and reduction in pain behaviors. Patients had continued to maintain their improvement at the 15-month follow-up. Arguably, the particular approach of therapy in this study falls outside the definition of couple therapy, although the intent was to change spousal behavior.

In an earlier study, Moore and Chaney (1985) reported on an out-patient couple group in which they investigated the effects of spousal involvement along with the patients in a 2-hour cognitive behavioral treatment program for eight sessions. Operant components of chronic pain were discussed and suggestions given to help the participants to rearrange their contingencies for pain and well behaviors. Control groups either received individual therapy or were wait-listed. The key hypothesis that attendance of spouses at the group therapy sessions would facilitate greater treatment gains and enhance the maintenance of these gains by promoting reinforcement for adaptive changes in patient's natural environment was not supported.

A noteworthy fact is that the studies involving spouses were not in the category of couple therapy, which usually involves the two partners together in the therapeutic process. As is evident, actual outcome studies dealing with couple therapy from a behavioral perspective are negligible and basically inconclusive. Reports of conjoint couple therapy for chronic pain are also very few.

An early retrospective clinical study of outcome of couple therapy with headache patients and their partners was reported by Roy (1989). This study investigated the factors that led to successful outcome of couple therapy for eight chronic headache patients and their partners. They were compared with eight couples who dropped out of therapy. Couples were evaluated using the MMFF. Specifically, the couples who successfully completed therapy were in less strifeful marriages and were confronted with specific life change events as opposed to the couples who dropped out, who gave evidence of serious marital strife. This was a very preliminary study to account for the factors that may predict positive couple therapy outcome for chronic headache sufferers.

Saarijarvi and his colleagues (1991, 1992), in a series of papers, have reported on the efficacy of couple therapy with chronic low-back pain (CLBP). They represent the only randomized controlled outcome studies of couple therapy for chronic pain. In their initial studies they reported their findings at the 1-year follow-up point. The findings were very encouraging and definitely established the benefits of couple therapy. In a subsequent study (Saarijarvi et al., 1992), they reported their findings at the 5-year follow-up point.

The most critical finding at the 5-year point was the maintenance of reduced psychological stress in the couple treatment group. During the same period, the distress level in the control patients increased. Significant difference between the treatment group and controls was observed in depression, anxiety, hostility, and obsessive-compulsive scores. Authors noted that a most significant finding was the decrease in the distress level in the couple treatment group. During the same period, the distress level in the control group actually rose. This was a critical finding as the most important obstacle to rehabilitation was emotional distress in CLBP patients. In their conclusion, authors suggested that the best results in the treatment of CLBP patients could be achieved by combining medical and interpersonal therapies before low-back pain became irreversible. On many psychological and social variables, CLBP patients share much in common with other chronic pain sufferers. Hence, an argument can be made in favor of couple therapy for chronic pain sufferers in general. However, this should not minimize the need for testing the efficacy of couple therapy with different chronic pain conditions.

Summary

Reports on couple therapy with the medically ill in general and with patients with chronic low-back pain in particular seem to indicate its overall efficacy in ameliorating relationship issues between couples. The issues that arise out of chronic illness and chronic pain may not be the same as the general relationship problems in otherwise healthy people. Our case illustrations and even research findings tend to show that there are direct consequences of chronic pain on interpersonal relationships as these couples experience some considerable changes in the way they need to organize their lives. Our older couple made that transition without a great deal of difficulty, whereas the younger couple were confronted with, what seemed like, impossible or even unacceptable changes. If one partner is unwilling to accept the limitations posed by chronic pain or illness in another partner, therapy may become a moot issue. Nevertheless, the weight of the evidence points in the direction that couple therapy for chronic pain sufferers may indeed be beneficial.

References

Backman, A., Haikonen, P., Hirvonen, E., et al. (1981) Chronic asthma in children: a medico-psychosocial approach. Psychiatrica Fennica (Suppl.): 85–95.

Barkley, B., Guevrenmont, D., Anastopoulos, A., et al. (1992) A comparison of three family therapy programs for treating family conflicts in adolescents with attention-deficit hyperactivity disorder. J. Consult. Clin. Psychol., 60: 450–462.

Baucom, D., Hahlweg, K., and Kuschel, A. (2003) Are waiting-list control groups needed in future marital therapy outcome studies? Behav. Ther., 34: 179–188.

Bjornstad, G. and Montgomery, P. (2006) Family therapy for attention deficit disorder or attention-deficit/hyperactivity disorder in children and adolescents. Cochrane Database Syst. Rev., Issue 1.

Brunk, M., Henggeler, S.W., and Whelan, J.P. (1987) Comparison of multisystemic therapy and parent training in the brief treatment of child abuse and neglect. J. Consult. Clin. Psychol., 55: 171–178.

Campbell, T. (2002) Physical disorders. In: Sprenkle, D. (Ed.) Effectiveness Research in Marriage and Family Therapy. Alexandria, VA, American Association of Marriage and Family Therapy.

Campbell, T. and Patterson, J. (1995) The effectiveness of family interventions in the treatment of physical illness. J. Marital Fam. Ther., 21: 545–583.

Carr, A. (2000) Evidence-based practice in family therapy and systemic consultation. J. Fam. Ther., 22: 273–295.

Chase, J. and Holmes, J. (1990) A two-year audit of a family therapy clinic in adult psychiatry. J. Fam. Ther., 12: 229–242.

Clark, M., Rubenach, S., and Winsor, A. (2003) A randomized controlled trial of an education and counseling interventions for families after stroke. Clin. Rehabil., 17: 703–712.

Clarkin, J., Carpenter, D., and Fertuck, E. (2003) The state of family therapy research. In: Sholevar, G. (Ed.) Family and Couples Therapy: Clinical Applications. Washington, DC, American Psychiatric Association.

Clarkin, J., Glick, I., Hass, G., et al. (1990) A randomized clinical trial of in-patient family intervention: results for affective disorders. J. Affect. Disord., 18: 17–28.

Crisp, A.H., Norton, K., Gowers, S., et al. (1991) A controlled study of the effect of therapies aimed at adolescent and family psychopathology in anorexia nervosa. Br. J. Psychiatry, 159: 325–333.

Cuijpers, P. (1999) The effects of family interventions on relatives' burden: a meta-analysis. J. Ment. Health, 8: 275–285.

Epstein, N. (2001) Cognitive-behavioral therapy with couples: empirical status. J. Cogn. Psychother., 15: 299–310.

Garrigan, J. and Bambrick, A. (1977) Family therapy for disturbed children: some experimental results in special education. J. Marriage Fam. Couns., 3: 83–93.

Guldner, C. (1990) Family therapy with adolescents. J. Group Psychother. Psychodrama Sociom., 43: 142–150.

Gustafsson, P.A., Kjellman, N.I., and Cederblad, M. (1986) Family therapy in the treatment of severe childhood asthma. J. Psychosom. Res., 30: 369–374.

Hagglund, K.J., Doyle, N.M., Clay, D.L., et al. (1996) A family retreat as a comprehensive intervention for children with arthritis and their families. Arthritis Care Res., 9: 35–41.

Henggeler, S.W. (1993) Multisystemic treatment of serious juvenile offenders: Implications for the treatment of substance abusing youths. In: Onken, L.S., Blaine, J.D., and Boren, J.J. (Eds.) Behavioral treatments for drug abuse and dependence: National Institute on Drug Abuse Research Monograph 137. Rockville, MD: NIH Publication No. 93-3684.

Johnson, S. (2002) Marital problems. In: Sprengle, D. (Ed.) Effectiveness research in marriage and family therapy. Washington, DC, American Association of Family Therapy.

Johnson, S. (2003) Couples therapy research: Status and directions. In: Sholevar, G. (Ed.) Textbook of Couples and Family Therapy. Washington, DC, American Psychiatric Association.

Keller, M. and Jost, R. (2003) Comprehensive counseling for families at risk for hereditary colorectal cancer: impact on perceptions and distress. Z. Med. Psychol., 12: 157–165.

Lask, B. and Matthew, D. (1979) Childhood asthma: a controlled trial of family psychotherapy. Arch. Dis. Child., 54: 116–119.

Lebow, J. and Gurman, A. (1995) Research assessing couple and family therapy. Annu. Rev. Psychol., 46: 27–57.

Leff, J., Vearnals, S., Brewin, C.R., et al. (2000) The London depression intervention trial. Randomized control trial of antidepressants vs couple therapy in the treatment and maintenance of people with depression living with a partner: clinical outcome and costs. Br. J. Psychiatry, 177: 95–100.

Lemmens, G., Verdegem, S., Heireman, S., et al. (2003) Helpful events in family discussion groups with chronic pain patients: a qualitative study of differences in perception between therapist/observers and patients/family members. Fam. Syst. Health, 21: 37–52.

Littell, J., Popa, M., and Forsythe, B. (2006) Multi-systemic family therapy for social, emotional, and behavioral problems in youth aged 10–17. Cochrane Database Syst. Rev., Issue 1.

Madanes, C. (1981) Strategic Family Therapy. San Francisco, CA.

Minuchin, S. (1974) Families and Family Therapy. Cambridge, MA, Harvard University Press, Jossey-Bass Publishers.

Moore, J. and Chaney, E. (1985) Out-patient group treatment of chronic pain: effects of spouse involvement. J. Consult. Clin. Psychol., 53: 326–334.

Olson, M. (2002) Clients' perceptions of the process of couple therapy: a qualitative and quantitative investigation. Dissertation Abstract International. Section B: The Science and Engineering, 62(12–b): 5975.

Priebe, S. and Sinning, U. (2001) Effects of brief couple therapy in cardiac rehabilitation: a controlled trial. Psychother. Med. Psychol., 51: 276–280.

Rivett, M. and Street, E. (2003) Family Therapy in Focus. London, Sage Publications.

Ro-Trock, G., Wellisch, D., and Schoolar, J. (1977) A family therapy outcome study in an inpatient setting. Am. J. Orthopsychiatry, 47: 514–522.

Roy, R. (1989) Couple therapy and chronic headache: a preliminary outcome study. Headache, 29: 455–457.

Roy, R. (2001) Social Relations and Chronic Pain. New York, Kluwer Academic/Plenum Publishers.

Roy, R. (2006) Chronic Pain and Family. New York, Springer.

Roy, R. and Frankel, H. (1995) How Good is Family Therapy. Toronto, University of Toronto Press.

Saarijarvi, S. (1991) A controlled study of couple therapy in chronic low-back patients: effects on marital satisfaction, psychological distress and health attitudes. J. Psychosom. Res., 35: 265–272.

Saarijarvi, S., Alanen, E., Rytokoski, U., and Hyyppa, M. (1992) Couple therapy improves mental well-being in chronic low-back patients: a controlled, five year study. J. Psychosom. Res., 36: 651–656.

Sack, P. and Thomasius, R. (2002) Effectiveness of family therapy and early intervention in drug misusing and drug dependent adolescents and young adults. Sucht: Zeitschrift für Wissenschaft und Praxis, 48: 431–438.

Satin, W., la Grece, A., Zigo, M., and Skyler, J. (1989) Diabetes in adolescence: effects of multi-family group intervention and parent simulation of diabetes. J. Pediatr. Psychol., 14: 259–275.

Sellers, T. (2000) A model of collaborative health care in out-patient medical oncology. Fam. Syst. Health, 18: 19–33.

Shadish, W. and Baldwin, S. (2003) The meta-analysis of MFT interventions. J. Marital Fam. Ther., 29: 547–570.

Sholevar, G. and Sahar, C. (2003) Medical family therapy. In: Sholevar, G. and Schwoeri, L. (Eds.) Family and Couples Therapy: Clinical Applications. Washington, DC, American Psychiatric Association.

Snyder, D., Castellani, A., and Whisman, M. (2006) Current status and future directions in couple therapy. Annu. Rev. Psychol., 57: 317–344.

Stanton, M., Todd, T., and Associates (1982) The Family Therapy of Drug Abuse and Addiction. New York, Guilford.

Stevenson, G. (1993) Combining quantitative and qualitative methods in evaluating a course of family therapy. J. Fam. Ther., 15: 205–224.

Szykula, S., Morris, S., Sudweeks, C., et al. (1987) Child-focused behavior and strategic therapies: outcome comparisons. Psychotherapy, 24: 546–551.

Thieme, K., Gromnica-Ihle, E., and Flor, H. (2003) Operant behavioral treatment of fibromyalgia: a controlled study. Arthritis Rheum., 49: 314–320.

Waring, E., Chamberlaine, C., Carver, C., et al. (1995) A pilot study of family therapy as a treatment for depression. Am. J. Fam. Ther., 23: 3–10.

Webster, L. (1992) Working with couples in a diabetics clinic: the role of the therapist in a medical setting. Sex. Marital Ther., 7: 189–196.

Yorke, J. and Shuldham, C. (2006) Family therapy for chronic asthma in children. Cochrane Database Syst. Rev., April (1): CD000089.

Chapter 4
Abuse, Chronic Pain and Psychodynamic Psychotherapy

Interest in any kind of a relationship between childhood abuse and pain dates back to the middle of the twentieth century. Engel (1959) wrote a seminal paper proposing a complex relationship between these two somewhat disparate phenomena. His theory of pain proneness, which was explored in depth by Roy (1998), has since received considerable empirical support. This chapter, to begin with, presents two cases where there was evidence of this relationship, followed by a brief review of the most recent empirical literature on abuse and pain. In this respect we review abuse and pelvic pain literature in some depth. In the final section we search for evidence of the effectiveness of psychotherapeutic interventions for these complex phenomena. We also review the literature on the use of psychodynamic psychotherapy in (1) various psychological and psychiatric disorders, (2) somatoform disorders, and (3) chronic pain.

Case Illustrations

We present two very different cases. The first story is that of Marion, a woman in her early forties who presented herself at the pain clinic with multiple pain problems. She was diagnosed with fibromyalgia. Treatment was less than effective and she lived with a high level of pain. In the course of routine psychosocial investigation, she revealed that she had been in a very abusive partner relationship. The marriage was over, but she continued to have "scars" from that relationship. Exploration of this relationship led to the revelation of her persistent sexual abuse by her biological father that commenced when she was 11.

The onset of this abuse coincided with the discovery of breast cancer in her mother. Her mother died a year later. Marion immersed herself in schoolwork and her father's reaction to the death of his wife seemed to be one of indifference. With the death of her mother the abuse stopped and she assumed the role of a surrogate wife and a mother to her younger brother. She left home to go to university at age 17. She never dated and led a very restricted life.

She completed her Masters program in English literature, which also coincided with her first significant relationship with a man. After a very short affair, he left without any explanation. Marion was lost and sought solace in God. She entered a

R. Roy, *Psychosocial Interventions for Chronic Pain*,
DOI: 10.1007/978-0-387-76296-8_4 © Springer Science+Business Media, LLC 2008

convent determined to leave the cruel and uncaring world behind her. She remained cloistered for 2 years and then entered a noncloistered convent. She stayed there another 2 years. She failed to find peace in the convents and continued to grieve the death of her mother and the breakup with her boyfriend.

She then married a very abusive man. She had known him during her university days. Initially, the marriage was satisfactory, but gradually her husband made increasing demands for sex. Marion was "disgusted" by these intimacies, but initially she just gave in. Later, she left him as his behavior became unpredictable and, at times, abusive. Finally, she got a divorce. It was in the process of discussing her disgust for physical intimacy that she began to recall her father's nightly visits to her bedroom and what ensued. She watched what this man was doing to her body from "up-above." It really was not happening to her, but to someone else. That is how she felt. This was the nature of her dissociative reaction. With her mother's rather sudden death, she had pushed the matter "to the back of her mind." It took Marion close to 2 months to unfold her story, which was followed by a prolonged period of grief. This was the first disclosure ever of her sexual abuse in the unlikely setting of a pain clinic. She stated somewhat poignantly that "How can you talk about something that you didn't even know happened."

Analysis

The most critical aspect of this case is Marion's attempt to wipe out her painful memories through dissociation and by later opting for a cloistered existence. Search for inner peace eluded her. "Something kept gnawing" inside her. During this period of her life she was pain free.

It is a matter of some curiosity that her pain problems began in earnest at the breakup of her marriage. The fact that she had a legitimate pain problem must be underscored. For the second time in her life she had somehow extricated herself from an abusive situation. Emotionally distraught and physically exhausted, she began her search for a cure to her pain problem. This was also the beginning of her social decline. A person raised in an upper-middle-class home with a graduate degree was now living in a rooming house on social assistance. She viewed her social decline with a degree of indifference that was hard to explain. It was as though she was doing penance for past misdeeds. Her futile efforts to run away from herself came to an end with her admission to the pain clinic. Her life had been filled with hurt and shame and guilt, and mostly unexpressed grief. The development of somatic symptoms when all other defense mechanisms fail is not a dramatic outcome. When she arrived at the pain clinic, Marion was more ready than ever to begin her backward journey that led to the rediscovery of her abuse, pain, shame, and betrayal by her parents, one for dying and the other for sexually violating her, followed by grief for her lost childhood. The clinical decision was that her unresolved childhood issues had to be properly addressed if she was to return to her potential. She was also treated for her pain, mainly with analgesics. The precise role her abuse played in the genesis of her pain problem is moot. What is undeniable was that she was far more disabled by her fibromyalgia than could be clinically accounted for. Hence, the significance of her childhood and marital abuse.

Marion remained in therapy for about 18 months. The approach was mainly psychodynamically oriented psychotherapy. We shall discuss its efficacy in the treatment of survivors of abuse. The rationale for adopting this particular approach was rooted in the recognition that she had to fully come to terms with the abuse, an experience she had chosen to bury deep into her psyche. This backward journey with all the accompanying pain was seen as an opportunity to rediscover her losses and emerge with a new understanding of herself, which would be devoid of guilt and shame and be supplanted by a clear understanding of her circumstances. At the point of termination, Marion had reintegrated back into the community and was actively working with a church organization. She had also found an apartment and literally started her life anew. Subsequently, she was discharged from the pain clinic.

Our next story is of a different type. Jean, a woman in her mid-twenties, presented with a history of inexplicable chronic pain, mainly in her chest and back; in this case there seemed to be more of a direct link between her pain and horrific physical and sexual abuse. During her first visit to the clinic, Jean was in a very heightened state of anxiety. She sat on the edge of her chair in a very taut position, rubbing her hands and speaking haltingly. Gradually, she revealed that she had grown up in a terrible home. Her mother was an alcoholic and her father was disabled with complications of diabetes. They argued and fought all the time. These were Jean's earliest memories. She recalled her childhood as being totally miserable and completely devoid of love and affection. She was terrified of abandonment by her parents. Her school years were altogether forgettable. She was a very poor student and was shunned by her peers. She could just about read and write and mathematics remained a total mystery to her.

Jean started associating with boys from a very early age and could not remember exactly at what age she became sexually active. At age 17 she formed a more permanent liaison with a man who was just slightly older than herself. She moved in with him after only a short acquaintance and for the following 2 years she was beaten, sodomized, and sexually abused. Any semblance of self-esteem she might have had just disappeared. The beatings she took usually involved him banging her head against a wall followed by pounding on her chest, which often left her with an open wound. He beat her without any provocation, but sometimes beatings followed her refusal to engage in anal sex, which she found excruciatingly painful.

These wounds resulted in several visits to the emergency department of her local hospital where she would usually be patched up. No one ever asked her about how she came to be so badly wounded. She never bothered to report him to the police mainly because of her fear of reprisal. The whole matter came to a dramatic end when on one occasion he produced a gun, threatening to kill her. A scuffle ensued and the gun went off, killing him. Following a major police inquiry, she was vindicated. This whole messy affair lasted some 2 years.

Jean further revealed that she was also sexually molested by her father. She was about 13 when the first incident occurred. She was alone in the house when her father called her over and put his hand inside her shirt. She fought him off, but he threatened that unless she cooperated he would beat her up. He also started supplying her with extra spending money and other material favors. She told her mother of his advances, but was not believed, and in fact she accused Jean of being responsible for encouraging him.

After the accidental death of her boyfriend, Jean's chest pain began in earnest, and thus began her journey through the maze of the healthcare system looking for a cure. Not until her visit to the pain clinic, Jean told us, had anyone inquired about her past. She was involved in another emotionally abusive relationship at the time of her admission to the pain clinic. She had made a vague suicidal gesture by swallowing a small amount of aspirin, which frightened her. Soon after this event her family physician referred her to a pain clinic.

The link between her chest pain and the father's sexual advances and the boyfriend's brutal beating in her upper torso, even from a symbolic point of view, cannot be easily ignored. Jean came from a poor and deprived background. She was intellectually and socially very constricted. She had few skills, and was seriously lacking in self-confidence. The communicative significance of her chest pain was nothing short of profound. Unfortunately, Jean failed to engage in psychotherapy and after an initial visit or two, she disappeared.

Abuse and Pelvic Pain: Empirical Support

In our previous review of this topic, we found that abuse was associated with varied medical conditions such as gastrointestinal disorders, premenstrual syndromes, eating disorders, and HIV infection (Roy, 1998). In this review of contemporary literature from 1999 to 2006 (April), we focus on abuse and pelvic pain and general chronic pain conditions. An association between chronic pelvic of unknown origin and early childhood abuse was noted by some of the early researchers searching for this association (Grossman, et al., 1981; Harrup-Griffiths et al., 1988; Walker et al., 1988). More recent research has refined some of the earlier findings. It should be noted that the etiologic significance of childhood abuse in the genesis of chronic pain remains somewhat moot.

Much more information has emerged about this relationship since the early studies. We present a selected review of the most recent literature on the topic of chronic pelvic pain (CPP) and childhood abuse. A number of studies have explored the complex nature of this relationship. Lampe and colleagues (2003) investigated the relationship between childhood abuse, stressful life events, and depression in 43 women with CPP and 40 female patients with chronic low-back pain (CLBP); 22 pain-free females served as control. A clear finding was that childhood physical abuse, stressful life events, and depression were generally associated with chronic pain, but childhood sexual abuse was strongly correlated with only pelvic pain. Besides, physical and sexual abuse during childhood showed a close relationship with an increased occurrence of stressful life events. So psychosocial factors must be taken into consideration in treating patients with chronic pain.

Thomas et al. (2006) explored the role of past abuse and suppression and repression of painful thoughts in a group of patients with CPP. They were compared with patients with endometriosis and a pain-free group. Suppression but not repression was related to higher levels of abuse and pain. Suppression of unwanted thoughts and emotions distinguished CPP patients from healthy controls. This study was a refinement of any simple association between CPP and childhood abuse, and showed the role of emotions in the expression of pain rather than abuse.

Similar challenges were evident in a study of trauma and dissociation in conversion disorder and CPP (Spinhoven et al., 2004). Their conclusion was that after controlling for psychopathology, in most cases the association of abuse with dissociation was not statistically significant. Hence, reliance on historical antecedents such as childhood abuse should be de-emphasized and more importance should be placed on recent potentially traumatizing events.

McGowan and associates (1998) conducted a meta-analysis to ascertain the psychological factors that were uniquely associated with CPP. Key words used for literature search were pelvic pain, chronic pelvic pain, sexual abuse, and physical abuse. The findings were complex. The results challenged the prevailing research findings of there being a consistent difference between women who had CPP without obvious pathology (normally associated with childhood abuse) and those with known pathology, on measures of psychological morbidity, depression, anxiety, neuroticism, and psychopathology. This study is of particular interest as the presence or absence of organic pathology may not predict the role of abuse in the presentation of CPP.

Nijenhuis and associates (2003) sought evidence for associations among somatoform dissociations, psychological dissociations, and reported trauma in patients with CPP. Fifty-two women with CPP whose pain had resisted treatment completed a set of standard questionnaires and were interviewed for DSM-IV dissociative disorders. The prevalence of a dissociative disorder was very low in this population. Women who reported more serious psychic trauma, in particular physical and sexual abuse, experienced more somatoform and psychological dissociation and trauma. Physical abuse/life threat posed by a person predicted somatoform dissociation best. The conclusion was that somatoform dissociation and reported trauma were strongly correlated phenomena. The significance of this study seems to be that idiopathic CPP may be a form of dissociative somatoform disorder. This is one plausible explanation for a selected group of CPP patients where the diagnosis is uncertain and there is clear evidence of significant physical and sexual abuse.

In a very important report Bergant and Widschwendter (1998) noted that the prevalence rate of CPP was found to be 15% in a large sample of women between the ages of 18 and 50 years. Any single cause of CPP was not found. Psychopathology as the main cause of CPP was reported to be suspect. However, frequent observation and the data on the relationship between CPP and psychological variables and physical and sexual abuse indicates that CPP may be a function of its association with other forms of abuse, particularly childhood sexual abuse. A multidisciplinary approach to treating these women was recommended.

Our last report was on a large-scale study to determine the prevalence and history of battering among 1780 women seeking general medical care (Diaz-Olavarrieta et al., 2002). Current physical and sexual abuse was reported by 152 women (9%). An identical number of women also reported abuse during pregnancy. Lifetime prevalence was 41%. Women with a current or past history of abuse reported more physical symptoms than did the nonabused group. Pelvic pain among other physical symptoms was frequent among the abused women.

This review indicates that although physical and sexual abuse may partly explain CPP, abuse may not be the only cause of this perplexing disorder. Second, both current and past abuse may be of equal significance. Psychopathology may underlie CPP at least in part of the population. The relative significance of physical vis-à-vis sexual abuse remains moot. In the following section we examine the broader literature on the relationship between chronic pain in general and physical and sexual abuse. Another point of note is that the actual rate of childhood abuse among CPP patients appears to be somewhat elusive.

Sexual and Physical Abuse and Chronic Pain Syndromes

Sound empirical evidence for a clear relationship between early abuse and chronic pain syndromes was relatively meager even during the 1990s. Two studies reported the rate of childhood abuse as 17% and 28%, respectively (Haber and Roos, 1985; Wurtle et al., 1990). These studies had a number of methodological shortcomings such as small sample sizes and simple correlational associations, which did not begin to explain any causal relationship between the two variables.

Finestone and colleagues (2000) examined healthcare utilization in 80 subjects. Of them, 26 subjects attended a group therapy program for persons with a history of child abuse, 33 were non-abused psychiatric patients, and 21 were nurses. Abused subjects reported a higher number of areas of pain in the body, more diffuse pain; also, there were more frequent diagnoses of fibromyalgia. They also reported having more surgeries, hospitalizations, and family physician visits. Clearly, abuse had far-reaching health consequences in these persons' adulthood as compared with psychiatric patients and normal persons.

One survey that is of particular interest examined the relationship between childhood abuse, current abuse, and a combination of both in 90 women between the ages of 18 and 82 who reported chronic pain (Green et al., 2001). Forty-three subjects reported a history of abuse. Of these, 12 cited childhood abuse, 12 adulthood abuse, and 14 repeated abuse.Subjects with a long-term history of abuse reported significantly higher number of pain and anxiety symptoms, and were more likely to report a history of substance abuse than those reporting childhood or adulthood abuse alone. The main conclusion was that there existed a clear association between history of abuse and health status.

A recent meta-analysis of the abuse and pain literature included retrospective reports of neglect and sexual or physical abuse experienced during childhood (Davis et al., 2005). Publications dates ranged from 1990 to 2001. Only studies involving a comparison group were selected. PubMed, Medline, and PschINFO were used to identify the relevant articles.

This review arrived at some convincing conclusions: (1) individuals who experienced childhood abuse or neglect also reported more pain symptoms and painful conditions than did the nonabused subjects; (2) patients with chronic pain were more likely to report childhood abuse than healthy controls; (3) patients with chronic pain were more likely to report childhood abuse than nonabused patients with chronic pain identified from the community; (4) individuals from the community reporting pain were more likely to report childhood abuse than individuals from the community not reporting pain. The conclusion was that childhood experience of abuse and neglect increased the risk of later life chronic pain as compared with individuals who were not abused. These conclusions again point to a relationship between childhood abuse and adult chronic pain, but they fail to explain the underlying cause for such a relationship. Theoretical explanations for this relationship were sought in the pathways by which adverse childhood experiences might influence the experience of chronic pain in adulthood. They may include emotional, physiological, psychological, and behavioral factors. A critical observation made by the authors was that reports of childhood abuse were linked with negative current life factors, including psychological distress, poor health behaviors, and abusive social relationships. And these factors, the authors proposed, may then be strongly linked to experience of pain symptoms. However, somatoform and dissociative disorders manifesting as chronic pain in adults have also been linked with childhood abuse.

Nevertheless, more recent research clearly points to the presence of such a relationship. However, not all studies confirm such a relationship. Albrecht (1998) investigated this relationship in a group of patients with fibromyalgia and chronic pain patients. His conclusion was that there did not exist any direct relationship or correlation between childhood abuse histories and the average dissociative experience reported by the two groups of patients. The weight of the overall evidence tends minimally to question that assertion.

Even this brief incursion into an examination of the relationship between abuse and pain leads to an unavoidable conclusion that abuse has a profound negative impact on health and consequently on healthcare utilization. The question that we shall presently address is, How effectively are chronic pain patients with a past or even current history of abuse treated when identified in a pain clinic setting?

Psychodynamic Psychotherapy and Abuse

Although Roy (1998) reported applying psychodynamic psychotherapy for treating many patients with a history of abuse and pain, empirical evidence for that intervention was, to say the least, weak. Reports on psychodynamic psychotherapy for survivors of childhood abuse during the period 1998–2006 are very few. On the contrary, other types of old and new interventions were reported during the same period. These included emotion-focused therapy (EFT) (Holowaty, 2005; Paivio, 2001; Paivio and Patterson, 1999; Paivio et al., 2001), skills training in affective and interpersonal regulations (STAIR) (Cahill et al., 2004), therapeutic alliance and negative mood regulation (Cloitre et al., 2004), and cognitive behavioral therapy (Cloitre et al., 2002).

The key question that arises in relation to therapy of abused patients with chronic pain is, How critical is it to treat the effects of abuse if the patient is to make a reasonable recovery? The answer is not known. The two case illustrations provided at the outset indicate that treating unresolved and/or ongoing abuse may be central to the treatment of these patients. Another point of note is that discovery of abuse in a pain clinic setting has to be a matter of chance, unless question of abuse is incorporated into routine psychosocial investigation. Our first case (Marion) responded well to treatment to the point that she resumed as close to a normal life as she had ever had. Our second patient, who was in a high-risk situation, dropped out. But had she stayed, our focus would have centered on her past and present abuse.

In treating Marion, we adopted a psychodynamic approach to the extent that the early focus of therapy was on the experiences of sexual abuse at the hands of her father and reliving those incomprehensible experiences to appreciate her helplessness, and to relieve her of some of the guilt that had colored her adult life so significantly. This kind of intervention is predicated on the assumption that patients' symptoms and problems are frequently meaningful creations, but the meaning may be more or less outside the awareness of the patients. This therapy involved helping Marion achieve awareness within the context of a safe and confiding relationship with the therapist.

It is noteworthy that Leichsenring (2003) in his review of empirical data derived from RCTs in support of psychodynamic psychotherapy was able to demonstrate its efficacy in the treatment of a wide variety of psychiatric disorders. Two other meta-analyses of the outcome literature, one for group therapy (DeJong and Gorey, 1996) and the other for individual psychotherapy (Price and Hilsenworth, 2001) for the treatment of survivors of childhood sexual abuse, have confirmed their efficacy.

We examine Price and Hilsenworth's (2001) article in some detail because it has direct relevance to the topic at hand. This analysis was based on eight articles and included four therapeutic approaches: (1) cognitive behavioral; (2) experiential; (3) psychodynamic–interpersonal; and (4) psychoeducational–supportive. The findings were positive along a number of important outcome measures. Individual intervention resulted in alleviation of psychiatric symptoms of depression and anxiety, less distorted thoughts, and improved interpersonal functioning, along with an alleviation of trauma-related symptoms. The authors pointed out that the studies they presented contained numerous strengths in terms of both efficacy and effectiveness. The studies selected were clearly defined with clear definitions of their target symptoms and valid measures. Treatment manuals were used in some of the studies. Nevertheless, they concluded that the literature remained incomplete as few studies provided a full description of the sample and failed to incorporate DSM-based diagnosis.

Because we used a psychodynamic approach to treat our patient, we examine it further. Price and Hilsenworth (2001) in their review of outcome literature of treatment of childhood abuse described psychodynamic and interpersonal therapies as placing an emphasis on the expression of affect and the exploration of relationship patterns in the etiology and maintenance of psychological disturbance.

Expressive and supportive techniques are incorporated in this method of therapy. They described one particular study of cognitive–analytic therapy, based on object relations theory, by Clark and Llewelyn (1994). This treatment was based on a manualized treatment program. The authors reported treating seven adult women who had reported childhood sexual abuse. Each patient received 16 sessions of therapy. The outcome revealed a reduction in depression, distorted beliefs, and other symptomatic distress after therapy.Posttreatment improvements were maintained at 3-month follow-up.

EFT, through a supportive therapeutic relationship, allows for the exploration of traumatic abuse memories. Paivio and Patterson (1999) observed that this intervention was embedded in an empathically responsive and collaborative relationship that provided safety and maximum client control over the process of therapy. This intervention was Gestalt-derived in which clients in their minds confronted their abusers. This intervention comes close to psychodynamic psychotherapy as it has in common the focus on the past and the centrality of the therapeutic relationship.

Pavaio and Nieuwenhuis (2000) reported on the effectiveness of EFT in treating 46 adult survivors of childhood abuse. Twenty-two of the subjects started therapy immediately and the remaining 24 received delayed treatment. Sexual abuse was reported by most subjects (11 in the treatment and 14 in the wait-group) in both groups. The inclusion of subjects was based on commonly accepted criteria for short-term, insight-oriented therapy, including motivation, the capacity to form a therapeutic relationship, and the capacity to focus on the circumscribed issue of child abuse. These inclusion criteria were derived from Malan (1979). Treatment consisted of 20-week individual psychotherapy. The research design was quasi-experimental. Attrition for the treatment group was 3 and for the wait-group 5.

The outcome was very positive on all psychological and psychiatric measures. The authors noted that EFT brought about statistically and clinically significant improvements for most clients in multiple domains of disturbance, including general and specific symptomatology, current abuse-related problems, global and specific interpersonal problems, and self-affiliation. Clients were maintaining these improvements in the 9-month follow-up. Clients in the delayed treatment showed minimal improvement over the wait-period, but after treatment showed improvements comparable to those of the immediate therapy group.

Summary

On the basis of this review, it can be stated with some level of confidence that the effectiveness of psychodynamic psychotherapy and its variants such as EFT was confirmed. The studies reviewed were characterized by sound methodology, but the actual number, only two, was very limited. Yet, the findings were very positive, and on that ground, an argument can be made for the use of this form of psychotherapy to treat survivors of abuse. To return to our cases, it would appear on reflection that despite pain issues, the history of abuse was of major significance, and at least in one case psychodynamic psychotherapy was applied with some success.

Somatoform Disorders and Psychodynamic Psychotherapy

Diagnosis of somatoform disorders among chronic sufferers is relatively common (Binzer et al., 2003; Novy et al., 2005; Türkcapar et al., 2005; Whalley and Oakley, 2003), as it is among persons with a history of abuse (Bass et al., 1999; Deseda-Smith, 1993; Fry, 1993; Kinzi et al., 1995; Loewenstein, 1990; Sansone et al., 2006). With these facts in mind, we conducted a literature search to find the application of psychodynamic psychotherapy with these patients.

In a unique article Nelson (2002) set out to investigate the nature of physical symptoms in sexually abused women. Somatization was the most common explanation offered for pain of unknown origin in patients with a history of sexual abuse. However, could the diagnosis of somatization overlook the presence of undetected injury and other pathophysiological conditions? The number of factors led her to question the adequacy of "somatization" as an explanation for the physical pain, the main concern being that the physical consequences of severe childhood abuse could inflict permanent physical damage leading to chronic pain. Nelson noted that many women who had resolved the emotional issues and improved their lives continued to have unexplained pain and debilitating symptoms. Many patients with a history of childhood abuse seen in pain clinics may fit this description. This article serves as a warning that although somatization remains the most accepted explanation for unexplained pain and physical symptoms in sexually abused women, this could lead to overlooking the underlying pathophysiology for the physical symptoms.

Some empirical support for Nelson's observations was reported in a study of 25 patients with psychogenic nonepileptic seizures (PNES), which have been associated with childhood abuse; they were compared with 33 controls with epilepsy on stressful life events and other risk factors for somatoform disorders (Tojek et al., 2000). Compared with control subjects, patients with PNES reported significantly more stressful negative life events, which also included adulthood abuse, and more current rumination, stress-related diseases, somatic symptoms, and only nominally more anxiety and depression. Many of these variables could be accounted for by stressful life events. This led the authors to conclude that PNES could be a response to a wide range of negative life events, including adulthood stressors, and may not be based on childhood abuse alone.

Our final report in this section investigates the relationships among Alexithymia, childhood abuse or trauma, and related vulnerability factors among chronic pain sufferers. A total of 16 women and 4 men were recruited from a university-based pain management center (Buckley, 1996). First and foremost, Alexithymia and current psychological distress were present in this population. Significantly, illness in a close relative during adulthood correlated positively and significantly with Alexithymia. Childhood abuse, chronic pain, and illness in a close family member combined with current psychological distress seemed to predict Alexithymia. This was an exploratory study.

Although somatoform disorder is not an uncommon diagnosis for unexplained chronic pain, and the empirical literature generally supports this link, evidence of relationship between childhood abuse and somatoform disorder (manifesting as chronic pain) is very sparse. This is a surprising omission, especially in view of ongoing findings of an as yet unexplained connection between childhood sexual abuse and pelvic pain. However, a few reports on the utilization of psychodynamic psychotherapy to treat somatoform (nonpain) disorders exist (Hamilton et al., 2000; Rudolf et al., 2004; Tritt et al., 1999; Zeek et al., 2003). These studies had one feature in common in that they all had a control group. We describe below the key findings of these studies.

We report Hamilton et al.'s (2000) study in some detail as it was an RCT to treat a group of patients with chronic functional dyspepsia (not necessarily a painful disorder, although some patients do complain of pain and discomfort) with brief psychodynamic–interpersonal psychotherapy. Treatment lasted for seven sessions, the first session lasting 3 hours. The rest of the sessions were 50 minutes long. Patients were assessed on a range of psychological functioning. The particular therapy used in this study was developed in England some 20 years ago and is manualized.

Ninety-five consecutive patients with chronic functional dyspepsia who had failed to respond to conventional medical intervention were randomly assigned to a treatment group consisting of 37 patients and 36 were assigned to a control group where they received supportive psychotherapy. All patients completed before and after self-report questionnaires 12 months later.

The results showed clear superiority of psychodynamic psychotherapy over supportive therapy with respect to patients' total symptom score; according to gatroenterologists, there were significant advantages for the psychodynamic psychotherapy group as compared with the control group. One year after treatment, symptomatic scores were similar. However, further analyses revealed that psychodynamic psychotherapy was superior, when patients with severe heartburn were excluded.

The authors concluded that this particular therapy may have both short-term and long-term benefits for patients with functional dyspepsia, but further research is called for. Cost-effectiveness of this therapy remains undetermined.

The following two studies were conducted in inpatient settings. Rudolf and colleagues (2004) reported on psychotherapy outcomes in a 5-year sample of patients suffering from anxiety and affective disorders and somatoform disorders. The treatment sample of 411 patients was compared with a control group of 312. The results were complex. Therapy effects, as measured by pre–post comparison of the patients' self-rating, were favorable, and especially noticeable in the anxiety and affective disorder patients. The effects for somatoform disorders were low, except that at follow-up, the rate of relapse was significantly higher in the anxiety and affective disorder group, and further improvement was observed in the somatoform group of patients. Overall, 80% of the patients reported satisfaction with psychodynamic psychotherapy.

In an investigation of the efficacy of psychotherapy, patients with anorexia nervosa were compared with patients suffering from somatoform disorders (not uncommon among chronic pain sufferers) (Zeek et al., 2003). Patients were drawn from day clinics and inpatient settings. Patients with anorexia nervosa with very low weight were preferentially treated in the inpatient setting. Somatoform patients in the inpatient group were also more affected. Therapeutic changes between the two settings were not significant. Both groups, however, showed significant improvement during the course of therapy. Psychotherapy, regardless of the severity of the disease(s) and settings, was demonstrated to be an effective form of intervention.

The final study in this section investigated a form of short-term psychotherapy based on transcultural psychology, which is purported to be in use in some 15 countries (Tritt et al., 1999). The initial results of one study designed to test the efficacy of this treatment involved 402 patients with psychiatric, psychosomatic, and somatic disorders. In a longitudinal study, patients treated with short-term psychotherapy showed a marked reduction in symptoms and a significant improvement in their feelings and behavior as compared with a control group. The control group failed to register any improvement. The results of a 5-year follow-up showed that the initial improvements reported by the patients upon completion of therapy were maintained. The authors claimed that this particular short-form psychotherapy produced long-term benefits.

Summary

The point of note about this group of studies is that chronic pain and/or abuse was not often the focus of studies reviewed. Only the first two studies had some connection to abuse (Buckley, 1996; Tojek et al., 2000), but these were not outcome studies. Yet, somatoform disorders are not at all uncommon in the chronic pain population and in the abused chronic pain population as witnessed by the abuse and pelvic pain literature. It is for this reason that we conducted this brief review to examine its effectiveness. Only an indirect conclusion can be drawn to the effect that chronic pain/abused patients presenting as suffering from somatoform disorder(s) may indeed benefit from psychodynamically oriented psychotherapy. However, any empirical evidence of successful outcome of psychotherapy for treating chronic pain patients with a history of abuse is yet to emerge.

Psychotherapy and Chronic Pain

A major review of the outcome literature on the efficacy of psychodynamic psychotherapy to treat a variety of disorders was reported by Leichsenring (2003). This review rectified one of the problems identified by Price and Hilsenworth (2001): DSM-IV diagnostic categories were used for the purpose of the review.

Bassett and Pilowsky (1984) reported on the efficacy of brief psychodynamic psychotherapy in treating chronic pain sufferers. Twenty-six patients attending a pain clinic in a large metropolitan area in Australia were randomly assigned to receive either 12 sessions of psychodynamic psychotherapy or 6 sessions of cognitively oriented supportive psychotherapy. Only a small proportion of patients attending the clinic were deemed suitable for this type of intervention as most patients were skeptical about the benefit of "talking" to deal with their pain.

Outcome measures included measures of depression, anxiety, and a global assessment of the patient's condition. The results were mixed. On the measures of depression and anxiety, no significant differences emerged between the two groups. On the global assessment, once again, the findings were nonsignificant. However, the authors carried out further analysis of the comments of the subjects, and found that within the supportive psychotherapy group only nine patients (22%) reported that they found the treatment useful in coping with pain. For the group provided with brief psychodynamic psychotherapy, positive experience was reported by 54% of the patients. This study had a number of methodological problems, the least of which was not the small number of subjects. The question of equivalency of treatments (6 sessions for one group and 12 sessions for another) employed in this study also arises. The results were also based on patients' subjective reporting. Nevertheless, the preliminary findings of this study laid the foundation for better-designed investigations to treat the efficacy of brief psychodynamic psychotherapy to treat chronic pain.

Irritable bowel syndrome (IBS) is a painful and chronic intestinal disorder, which has remained somewhat impervious to treatment even to date. There is a general recognition that psychosocial factors influence this disorder, but at the time that this study was undertaken there was very little attention paid to adopting a comprehensive medical and psychosocial approach to treating this disease. A number of RCTs have established the effectiveness of psychodynamic psychotherapy for IBS, potentially a very painful disorder (Creed et al., 2003; Guthrie et al., 1991; Svedlund, 1983). Treatment in all three studies involved brief therapies, which are discussed in Chapter 7. Subjects in these studies were not abused. Treatment for this condition, however, remains a challenge.

Emotional and physical abuse among the IBS sufferers is said to be common (Ali et al., 2000; Lesserman et al., 1996; Walker et al., 1995). However, the notion of a linkage between abuse and IBS remains controversial (Talley et al., 1995). Keefer and Blanchard (2001) summarized the mechanism proposed by the supporters of such a relationship by suggesting that abuse (1) reduces the threshold of gastrointestinal symptom experience or increases intestinal motility; (2) modifies one's appraisal of bodily sensations through an inability to control symptoms; and (3) leads to feelings of guilt and internal responsibility, making disclosure of symptoms unlikely. Our search failed to find any empirical study utilizing psychodynamic psychotherapy to treat IBS patients with a history of abuse.

There exists only one report of an RCT for the efficacy of psychodynamic psychotherapy for treating chronic pain (Monsen and Monsen, 2000). For this reason alone, we report its findings in some detail. The sample was selected from an employee group at a large Norwegian office company. In 1994, 160 subjects with pain complaints were all self-referred to the company's own health service. They were offered the opportunity of participating in a treatment study involving psychodynamic body therapy (PBT). PBT is a combination of a particular form of dynamic psychotherapy and physical therapy designed to accelerate the psychotherapeutic process. Patients were divided into two randomized groups of 20 each. Matching was done separately for men and women. Outcome assessments utilizing a host of psychological measures were conducted prior to the implementation of therapy and at the termination of therapy and at 1-year follow-up. The treatment group received 33 sessions of PBT and the other half received treatment as usual (TAU).

The results were impressive. The differences between groups were significant on the measures both at T2 and at T3. The largest changes were achieved during therapy. In broad terms, this study showed that at T2 the pain was significantly reduced in the PBT group as compared with controls, and a full 50% of the patients reported being pain-free. They also reported significant changes on levels of somatization, depression, anxiety, denial, assertiveness, and social withdrawal. These results remained stable at T3 and some of the PBT patients continued to improve even beyond T3.

A few points about this study are noteworthy. First, the population, all employees in a firm, was significantly different from the pain population generally encountered in pain clinics. Pain clinic populations are generally far more disabled by their pain than the study population. The fact that the subjects in this study were employed full-time sets them apart from the clinical chronic pain population.

The second point of note is the therapy itself. It is a hybrid form, combining psychological and physical therapies as a unique form of psychotherapy. The therapy was provided by a clinical psychologist who was also a trained physical therapist. This has to be viewed as a rare combination of training and skills, and may not be readily available in a pain clinic setting. However, the authors do refer to training therapists in this model who were involved in another study involving patients with fibromyalgia. Nevertheless, an average pain clinic in North America may be at a disadvantage in implementing this model of intervention that requires complex training for the therapists.

Summary

To state the obvious, only two studies reported on the effectiveness of psychotherapy for chronic pain conditions. One of the studies investigated its effectiveness with IBS and the other with general chronic pain complaints in a community setting. Findings were positive in both studies. However, the degree to which the subjects in the study may share some of the well-known characteristics of pain clinic attendees in terms of their disability, for example, is not clear. It should also be noted that psychodynamic psychotherapy is rarely a treatment of choice in pain clinic settings where cognitive behavioral interventions dominate.

Conclusion

The rationale for psychodynamic psychotherapy as the treatment of choice for patients with chronic pain with a history of childhood abuse lends itself to common sense. Despite the limited number of studies, the results are encouraging. If issues of childhood abuse in chronic pain sufferers are predominant and must be treated, a case can be made for its use. Overall, both clinical and empirical evidence for the use of psychodynamic psychotherapy for treating this group of patients remain wanting.

References

Albrecht, W. (1998) Dissociation, childhood trauma, locus of control and coping style among fibromyalgia and other chronic pain patients. Dissertation Abstracts International. Section B: The Sciences and Engineering, 58(11-B).

Ali, A., Toner, B., Stuckless, N., et al. (2000) Emotional abuse, self-blame, and self-silencing in women with irritable bowel syndrome. Psychosom. Med., 62: 76–82.

Bass, C., Bond, A., Gill, D., and Sharpe, M. (1999) Frequent attenders without organic disease in a gastroenterology clinic: patients characteristics and health care use. Gen. Hosp. Psychiatry, 21: 30–38.

Bassett, D. and Pilowsky, I. (1984) A study of brief psychotherapy for chronic pain. J. Psychosom. Res., 29: 259–264.

Bergant, A. and Widschwendter, M. (1998) Chronic pelvic pain: gynecologic and psychosocial factors. Arch. Womens Ment. Health, 1: 103–108.

Binzer, M., Almay, B., and Eisemann, M. (2003) Chronic pain disorder associated with psychogenic versus somatic factors: a comparative study. Nord. J. Psychiatry, 57: 61–66.

Buckley, E. (1996) Alexithymia, childhood abuse/trauma, and psychosomatic vulnerability in chronic pain patients. Dissertation Abstract International. Section B: The Science and Engineering, 57(5-B): 3403.

Cahill, S.P., Zoellner, L.A., Feeny, N.C., and Riggs, D.S. (2004) Sequential treatment for child abuse-related posttraumatic stress disorder: methodological comment on Cloitre, Koenen, Cohen, and Han (2002). J. Consult. Clin. Psychol., 72: 543–548.

Clark, S. and Llewelyn, S. (1994) Personal constructs of survivors of childhood abuse receiving cognitive analytic therapy. Br. J. Med. Psychol., 67: 273–289.

Cloitre, M., Koenen, Cohen, L., and Han, H. (2002) Skills training in affective and interpersonal regulation followed by exposure: a phase based treatment for PTSD related to childhood abuse. J. Consult. Clin. Psychol., 70: 1067–1074.

Cloitre, M., Chase-Stovell, K., Miranda, R., and Chemtob, C. (2004) Therapeutic alliance, negative mood regulation, and treatment outcome in child abuse related post-traumatic stress disorder. J. Consult. Clin. Psychol., 72: 411–416.

Creed, F., Fernandes, L., Guthrie, E., et al. (2003) The cost-effectiveness of psychotherapy and paroxetine for severe irritable bowel syndrome. Gastroenterology, 124: 303–317.

Davis, D., Luecken, L., and Zautra, A. (2005) Are reports of childhood abuse related to the experience of chronic pain in adulthood? A meta-analytic review of the literature. Clin. J. Pain, 21: 398–405.

DeJong, T. and Gorey, K. (1996) Short-term versus long-term group work with female survivors of childhood sexual abuse: a brief meta-analytic review. Soc. Work Groups, 19: 19–27.

Deseda-Smith, D. (1993) Sexual abuse and somatic complaints in female psychiatric inpatients. Dissertation Abstract International, 53(9-A): 3107.

Diaz-Olavarrieta, C., Ellertson, C., Paz, F., et al. (2002) Prevalence of battering among 1780 outpatients at an internal medicine institution in Mexico. Soc. Sci. Med., 55: 1589–1602.

Engel, G. (1959) Psychogenic pain and the pain-prone patient. Am. J. Med., 26: 899–918.

Finestone, H., Stenn, P., Davies, F., et al. (2000) Chronic pain and health care utilization in women with a history of childhood sexual abuse. Child Abuse Negl., 24: 547–556.

Fry, R. (1993) Adult physical illness and childhood sexual abuse. J. Psychosom. Res., 89–103.

Green, C., Flowe-Valencia, H., Rosenblum, L., and Tait, A. (2001) The role of childhood and adulthood abuse among women presenting for chronic pain management. Clin. J. Pain, 17: 359–364.

Grossman, R., Doerr, H., Caldiorla, D., et al. (1981) Borderline syndrome and incest in chronic pelvic pain patients. Int. J. Psychiatry Med., 10: 79–86.

Guthrie, E., Creed, F., Dawson, D., and Tomenson, B. (1991) A controlled trial of psychological treatment of irritable bowel syndrome. Gastroenterology, 100: 450–457.

Haber, J. and Roos, C. (1985) Effects of spouse and/or sexual abuse in the development and maintenance of chronic pain in women. Adv. Pain Res. Ther., 9: 889–895.

Hamilton, J., Guthrie, E., Creed, F., et al. (2000) A randomized control trial of psychotherapy in patients with chronic functional dyspepsia. Gastroenterology, 119: 661–669.

Harrup-Griffiths, J., Katon, W., Walker, E., et al. (1988) The association between chronic pelvic pain, psychiatric diagnosis, and sexual childhood abuse. Obstet. Gynecol., 171: 589–594.

Holowaty, K. (2005) Process characteristics of client-identified helpful events in emotion-focused therapy for adult survivors of childhood abuse. Dissertation Abstract International. Section B: The Sciences and Engineering, 65(7-B).

Keefer, L. and Blanchard, E.B. (2001) The effects of relaxation response meditation on the symptoms of irritable bowel syndrome results of a controlled treatment study. Behav. Res. Ther., 39(7): 801–811.

Kinzi, J., Traweger, C., and Biebl, W. (1995) Family background and sexual abuse associated with somatization. Psychother. Psychosom., 64: 82–87.

Lampe, A., Doering, S., Rumpold, G., et al. (2003) Chronic pain syndrome and their relation to childhood abuse and stressful life-events. J. Psychosom. Res., 54: 361–367.

Leichsenring, F. (2003) Are psychodynamic and psychoanalytic therapies effective? Int. J. Psychoanal., 86: 841–868.

Lesserman, J., Drossman, D., Li, Z., Toomey, T., Nachmann, G., and Glogau, L. (1996) Sexual and physical abuse history in gastroenterology practice: how types of abuse impact health status. Psychosom. Med., 58: 4–15.

Loewenstein, R. (1990) Somatoform disorders in victims of incest and child abuse. In: Kluft, R. (Ed.) Incest Related Syndromes of Adult Psychopathology (pp. 75–111). Washington, DC: American Psychiatric Association.

Malan, D. (1979) Individual Psychotherapy and the Science of Psychotherapy. London, Butterworths.

McGowan, L., Clark-Carter, D., and Pitts, M. (1998) Chronic pelvic pain: a meta-analytic review. Psychol. Health, 13: 937–951.

Monsen, M. and Monsen, T. (2000) Chronic pain and psychodynamic body therapy. Psychotherapy, 37: 257–269.

Nelson, S. (2002) Physical symptoms in sexually abused women: somatization or undetected injury. Child Abuse Rev., 11: 51–64.

Nijenhuis, E., van Dyck, R., ter-Kuile, M., et al. (2003) Evidence for association among somatoform dissociation, psychological dissociation and reported trauma in patients with chronic pelvic pain. J. Psychosom. Obstet. Gynaecol., 24: 87–98.

Novy, D., Berry, M., Palmer, L., et al. (2005) Somatic symptoms in patients with chronic non-cancer related and cancer-related pain. J. Pain Symptom Manage., 29: 603–612.

Paivio, S. and Patterson, L. (1999) Alliance development in therapy for resolving child abuse issues. Psychotherapy, 36: 343–354.

Paivio, S. and Nienwenhuis, J. (2000) Efficacy of emotional focused therapy for adult survivors of child abuse. J. Traumatic Stress, 14: 115–134.

Paivio, S. (2001) Stability of retrospective self-report of child abuse and neglect before and after therapy abuse issues. Child Abuse Negl., 25: 1053–1068.

Paivio, S., Hall, I., Holowaty, K., et al. (2001) Imaginal confrontation for resolving child abuse issues. Psychother. Res., 11: 433–453.

Price, J. and Hilsenworth, M. (2001) A review of individual psychotherapy outcome for adult survivors of childhood sexual abuse. Clin. Psychol. Rev., 21: 1095–1121.

Roy, R. (1998) Childhood Abuse and Chronic Pain: A Curious Relationship? Toronto, University of Toronto Press.

Rudolf, V., Jacobsen, T., Micka, R., and Schumann, E. (2004) Results of psychodynamic in-patient psychotherapy in relation to diagnosis. Z. Psychosom. Med. Psychother., 50: 37–52.

Sansone, R., Pole, M., Dakroub, H., and Butler, M. (2006) Childhood trauma, borderline personality symptomatology, and psychophysiological and pain disorders in adulthood. Psychosomatics, 47: 158–162.

Spinhoven, P., Roelofs, K., Moene, F., et al. (2004) Trauma and dissociation in conversion disorder and chronic pelvic pain. Int. J. Psychiatry Med., 34: 305–318.

Svedlund, J. (1983) Psychotherapy in irritable bowel syndrome: a controlled study. Acta Psychiatr. Scand., 67: 77–86.

Talley, N., Fett, S., and Zinsmeister, A. (1995) Self-reported abuse and gastrointestinal disease in outpatients: association with irritable bowel-type symptoms. Am. J. Gastroenterol., 90: 366–371.

Thomas, E., Moss-Morris, R., and Faquhar, C. (2006) Coping with emotions and abuse history in women with chronic pelvic pain. J. Psychosom. Res., 60: 109–112.

Tojek, T., Lumley, M., Barkley, G., Mahr, G., and Thomas, A. (2000) Stress and other psychosocial characteristics of patients with psychogenic nonepileptic seizures. Psychosomatics, 41: 221–226.

Tritt, K., Loew, T., Meyer, M., Werner, B., and Peseschian, N. (1999) Positive psychotherapy: effectiveness of an inter-disciplinary approach. Eur. J. Psychiatry, 13: 231–234.

Türkcapar, H., Özyurt, F., Örsel, S., and Türkcapar, F. (2005) Psychiatric morbidity in patients with pain and unexplained symptoms. Pain Clinic, 17: 289–295.

Walker, E., Gelfand, A., Gelfand, M., and Katon, W. (1995) Psychiatric diagnosis and physical victimization, and disability in patients with irritable bowel syndrome. Psychol. Med., 25: 1259–1267.

Walker, E., Katon, W., Harrup-Griffthis, J., et al. (1988) Relationship of chronic pelvic pain to psychiatric diagnosis and childhood sexual abuse. Am. J. Psychiatry, 150: 1502–1506.

Whalley, M. and Oakley, D. (2003) Psychogenic pain: a study using multidimensional scaling. Contemp. Hypnosis, 20: 16–24.

Wurtle, S., Kaplan, G., and Keairnes, M. (1990) Childhood sexual abuse among chronic pain patients. Clin. J. Pain, 6: 110–113.

Zeek, A., Scheidt, C., Hartmann, A., and Wirsching (2003) In-patient psychotherapy or partial hospitalization? Psychotherapeut, 48: 420–425.

Chapter 5
Interpersonal Psychotherapy

This chapter presents two cases and theoretical and empirical justification for the use of interpersonal psychotherapy (IPT) in treatment. We shall first present the case of Lisa, an adolescent, followed by a literature review and then the case of Clara, a middle-aged woman with a complicated medical history. Lisa, a young teenager, had hysterectomy and vaginoplasty in her preteen years and continued to experience severe and persistent abdominal pain. Apart from the pain, these surgeries had a profound impact on the patient, her parents, and to a lesser degree on her only older brother. Collectively, they were all in a state of mourning. Over time, they were able to articulate their grief as centering on Lisa's infertility. Lisa had a sense of being different, but the fact that she could not conceive was somewhat theoretical for her. Yet, she felt different from the other kids. Lisa was referred to a pain clinic by her pediatrician who had exhausted all means of pain control for this young person, who suggested that a psychotherapeutic approach may prove beneficial.

This family had emigrated to Canada from South America when the children were infants. Lisa's parents were deeply religious. Lisa shared her parents' values and had come to believe that her serious illness and the subsequent surgeries, which had left her permanently scarred, were divine retribution for something or other. She was altogether unsure about her perceived punishment, for she had always been a good person and followed her parents' guidance.

Lisa had no sense of belonging, which is especially serious for a young teen, with her peers at school. She had a strong feeling of being different from her peers. While she was in hospital, several children she had come to know died. She was surrounded by seriously ill children. She felt that her illness had robbed her of her childhood and she had grown up too fast. Her peers at school seemed preoccupied with superficial things like clothes and boys. She had time for neither. Her mother was her best friend.

What did Lisa think about her surgeries? Her immediate response was that for one thing she would never have any children. She questioned why she should be deprived so. The operations had left her feeling less than a female when she was almost on the verge of womanhood. Her parents never talked about it, but she knew that they were disappointed. Was all this making her sad? Sometimes she cried, but always made sure that no one was around. She did not feel very attractive. She did not like her own looks. Perhaps that was the reason, Lisa speculated, that no one liked her at school.

R. Roy, *Psychosocial Interventions for Chronic Pain*,
DOI: 10.1007/978-0-387-76296-8_5 © Springer Science+Business Media, LLC 2008

Lisa drew a picture of her predicament. The picture was entirely black showing a blob in the middle surrounded by thick black walls. She explained that the blob in the middle was Lisa, and she had no way out. This was a telling portrayal of her self-image—a person imprisoned and without a future. Did the picture have anything to do with the loss of her uterus? That was part of it, but she had this overwhelming feeling of being alone. She was also the cause of much rift between her parents. She had overheard them arguing about her. They had hardly ever argued before she got sick.

A threat, a challenge, a blow—all these terms can be interchangeably used to describe Lisa's feelings about herself. She had been irrevocably changed. This happened at a critical phase of her development when her sense of womanhood was just beginning to take root. Her conflict around her peer relations manifested as both wanting and not wanting to be part of her peer group, making her feel unattractive. They confirmed her sense of being different as well as bad. In her mind Lisa tried to fight the loss of her reproductive organs by trying to minimize it. She could adopt not one but many children when she grew up, and she would like to be a pediatrician and help sick children.

However, just beneath the surface was the overwhelming feeling of having been cheated of her womanhood, letting down her family, and surely being different than her peers—who she thought were all better-looking than her, and yet still had their uterus intact. Psychological effects of hysterectomy on women can be quite negative, and there is consensus that many women regard this surgery as a threat to their core female identity (Roy, 2004). These responses vary based on age, personality, personal circumstances, and so on.

For a young teenager, this particular loss is likely to have considerable poignancy. Unfortunately, the literature is silent on this topic and there is always a risk of drawing too many generalized conclusions based on a single case. What, however, is undeniable is that Lisa's emerging sexual identity was under severe strain. Curiously, she never asked the question of "Why me?" Rather, she viewed this as divine retribution for reasons that were far from self-evident. This perspective only added to her heightened sense of guilt and "badness." Self-recrimination was the driving force. Lisa was in a state of mourning. She was taken into therapy, and over time made significant gains.

The collective response of her parents and brother to the surgeries was great sadness. This had serious consequences for our young patient, and contributed to her feelings of guilt. Her mother tried to maintain a very positive attitude, and was indeed our patient's main source of support. From time to time, though, even the mother succumbed to despair, depression, and guilt over her daughter's loss of reproductive organs. The entire family system was in the throes of grief, and this had gone on for quite some time. Our approach to deal with this loss was to persuade the family to consider the reasons behind the surgeries and what the consequences might have been without them. Somehow, this simple reality was buried under their overwhelming sense of loss and grief, complicated as it was by guilt.

Lisa's critical developmental stage, the family's reaction to her surgeries, their collective belief in divine retribution, and the very nature of the loss, namely, her ability to ever have babies, contributed to making this situation very grievous indeed. Another fact of some import is that the separation–individuation process in adolescents with chronic illness ceases to be a smooth process, and in general terms, it is slowed down. The difficulties caused by the illness and the interaction between the illness, on the one hand, and the process of adolescence, parents, social class, ethnicity, and culture, on the other hand, profoundly impact on this process. Lisa unquestionably was in the throes of such a struggle, which was complicated by her parents' religious beliefs and her dependence, of necessity, on her mother.

Lisa's psychotherapy was based largely on the principles of IPT, with its focus on significant life events, grief, and her self-image (Ravitz, 2006; Tsi-Wai Chan, 2005; Weissman et al., 2000). IPT is a short-term psychotherapy lasting between 12 and 16 weeks. Several manuals are available for IPT (Mufson et al., 2004; Stuart and Robertson, 2003). IPT focuses on interpersonal problems rather than on intrapsychic or cognitive aspects. Its major attraction is that it uses a biopsychosocial model, which is also the model in wide use in the treatment of chronic pain. Grief, interpersonal role disputes, role transitions, and loneliness or social isolation are the key components of intervention. Therapy has three phases: beginning, middle phase and the focal problem areas, and the end therapy.

The extent to which Lisa was affected by all these four areas was quite uncanny. It is also noteworthy that IPT has been shown to be effective in treating adolescents with depression (Mufson et al., 2006). Lisa's depression varied between mild and moderate. She had good and bad days, often determined by her pain levels. IPT was modified to the extent that therapy lasted longer than the prescribed number of sessions and hence could not be considered strictly short term.

In therapy, Lisa gave up her preoccupation with the loss of her uterus. She began to show concerns that were more congruent with those of a teenager. She insisted that she was too young to have a boyfriend, but she got along with boys just fine. A major shift in her attitude toward her peers also began to emerge. She was not so judgmental about them. Nor did she feel herself excluded by them. She had a small group of close friends, but got along well with her schoolmates. She simply ceased to see herself as an outsider. Her grades improved, and she began to have serious thoughts about pursuing a medical career. She remained concerned about her appearance. Efforts were made to see her on a weekly basis, but due to the up-and-down nature of her pain and the other commitments she had, it was somewhat more sporadic. Lisa remained in active therapy for about 6 months and was kept under review for an indefinite period. Although her psychological and social functioning significantly improved, her pain (which was being treated medically mainly with analgesics) remained somewhat impervious to treatment.

Adolescent Chronic Pain and Psychosocial Issues

First and foremost, it is critical to recognize that chronic pain problems in adolescents are capable of producing serious quality-of-life issues and problems. Merlijn and associates (2006) in their study of 194 adolescents between the ages of 12 and

18 with problems of chronic pain showed that pain intensity and vulnerability contributed significantly and uniquely to the variance of most quality-of-life domains. Their analysis revealed that psychosocial variables accounted for a significant variance in the adolescents' quality of life, even when controlling for pain variables.

An earlier study of 222 adolescents and 144 controls with chronic pain by Merlijn and associates (2003) found that the chronic pain group was more vulnerable in terms of neuroticism, negative fear of failure, and less social acceptance. Their analysis of the contribution of psychosocial factors to chronic pain sustained the positive relation between vulnerability, (less) pain reinforcement, pain models, and the ability to cope with pain.

Weel and colleagues (2005) noted that instruments for measuring pain-related problems in adolescents were few and far between, especially based on personal experiences of the adolescents. One twenty-nine adolescents with chronic pain without documented physical etiology problems completed a 57-item problem list, which was based on interviews with a similar group of adolescents. Their analysis yielded four domains: (1) concentration; (2) mobility; (3) adaptability; and (4) mood. They recommended further research to validate their instrument. Even this limited review indicates that the problems adolescents are likely to encounter because of chronic pain tend to bear a strong resemblance to Lisa's problems prior to the onset of therapy.

Psychological treatment literature for adolescent pain is summarized in the following study. The conclusions were mixed in a major meta-analytic review of the psychosocial therapy literature for its effectiveness in treating chronic pain in young persons (Eccleston et al., 2002). Eighteen articles on the outcome of psychosocial therapy for chronic pain in children met the stringent criteria for this analysis. A vast majority of these articles reported on behavioral and cognitive behavioral interventions. A strong case was made for treating children as a matter of routine with chronic headache using behavioral and cognitive behavioral interventions.

Although mainly relaxation and cognitive behavioral therapy for treating chronic pain in children were found to be very effective, this was less so as far as improvement in mood, function, or disability associated with chronic pain was concerned. This is an important point to be noted in the context of the choice of treatment for Lisa. She had experienced a major trauma that had serious emotional and interpersonal consequences. A treatment paradigm was sought that would effectively address those issues. As noted earlier, IPT was the therapy of choice.

Effectiveness of IPT

Loss and grief is ubiquitous in the chronic pain population (Roy, 2004, see chapter 5). Loss of job, family roles, social activities, and a host of other normal human activities are put in jeopardy by chronic pain. To some degree these problems are evident in both our cases. Depressive symptoms are ubiquitous in this population. IPT, with its focus on negative life events, depression, and disruption of interpersonal relations, would appear to be particularly well suited to treat chronic pain sufferers with issues of loss and interpersonal conflicts.

Research evidence in support of IPT is impressive. The comprehensive reviews of Weissman et al. (2000) and Stuart and Robertson (2003) testify to that. The now famous study conducted by the National Institute of Mental Health, which is still regarded as the gold standard for psychotherapy efficacy research, confirmed that IPT was superior to placebo and equal to CBT and imipramine for mild to moderate depression. A study by Elkin and colleagues (1989) randomized acutely depressed patients to IPT, CBT, and imipramine and clinical management. The Hamilton Rating Scale for Depression was used to measure the levels of depression. On that scale IPT was found to be superior to placebo and equal to imipramine for mild to moderate depression. IPT was slightly more superior to CBT for severe depression. Altogether, 55% of patients who completed IPT achieved remission of depression.

However, Klein and Ross's (1993) reanalysis of Elkin et al.'s (1989) data led to a different conclusion, namely, treatment with medications was superior to psychotherapies, and the psychotherapies were somewhat superior to placebo. Effects were more pronounced among the more symptomatic and impaired patients. Despite this finding to the contrary, the NIMH study continues to be regarded as groundbreaking.

Several recent studies have attested to the effectiveness of IPT (deMello et al., 2005; Kotova, 2005; Leibing et al., 2005; Salsman, 2006). deMello and colleagues conducted a systematic review. They selected RCTs from all available databases from 1974 to 2002. Thirteen studies fulfilled the inclusion criteria and four meta-analyses were performed. The efficacy of IPT proved superior to placebo, similar to medication, and did not improve when combined with medication. Overall, IPT was superior to CBT. Their conclusion was that IPT was an efficacious psychotherapy for depressive spectrum disorders and may be superior to some other manualized psychotherapies.

Kotova (2005) conducted a meta-analysis of short-term IPT to estimate its efficacy at posttreatment and at follow-up. The sample in the studies consisted of physically healthy adult women diagnosed with depression or suffering from eating disorders and being treated as outpatients. The efficacy of IPT when compared with no treatment was estimated to be in the range of 0.60–0.73 effect sizes, depending on the outcome measures chosen by the original researchers. Minimum treatment such as only educational input compared with IPT produced effect sizes in the range of 0.37–0.48. The author concluded that in terms of relative efficacy, the meta-analysis confirmed that compared with other established psychological therapies, IPT was not convincingly superior. The combination of IPT and medication was not superior to each treatment alone. IPT, however, retained some of its efficacy at follow-up. This conclusion was strong in relation to eating disorders. This study, while finding IPT to be an effective, although with qualification, form of psychotherapy, somewhat deviated from deMello et al.'s (2005) very positive findings.

Leibing and his colleagues' (2005) review has limited relevance to our topic. They reviewed literature on the efficacy of short-term psychodynamic psychotherapy (STPP), which also included IPT. The effect sizes of STPP were compared with those of WLCs, of the usual treatments, and of other forms of psychotherapies. STPP yielded significant pre–post effect size, which increased at follow-up. STPP was superior to WLCs and as usual treatments, but no differences emerged between STPP and other forms of psychotherapy. However, the outcome of ITP was only one component of this review that requires modification of any exaggerated claims of the efficacy of IPT alone. Salsman (2006) tested the efficacy of time-limited interpersonal psychotherapy (TLIPT) to determine whether TLIPT was capable of both symptom changes and interpersonal changes. A sample of 61 clients who identified interpersonal problems as a primary problem were treated with 9–16 sessions of TLIPT. Her analysis clearly revealed that clients experienced significant reductions in measures of symptoms and interpersonal distress. Clients exhibited an increase in friendliness and a decrease in hostility. They also showed an increase in dominance and a decrease in submissiveness. Virtually on all measures of relationships, clients showed measurable improvement. These reviews taken together, although varying in details, tend to confirm the overall efficacy of IPT. The question of whether IPT is superior to other forms of psychotherapies may be considered moot.

IPT to treat chronic pain is a hugely underresearched area. Our search produced two articles. The first was a major study involving 189 subjects aged 69 years and above with complaints of body pain and depression (Karp et al., 2005). Investigation centered on the influence of body pain on (1) time to treatment response and (2) suicidal ideation in late-life depression. Treatment consisted of paroxetine upto 40 mg daily and a minimum of 10 weekly IPT sessions before ending the acute treatment and the continuation phase of the study. Patients received ten sessions of IPT before being randomized in the maintenance phase of the protocol. Depression was measured by the Hamilton Rating Scale for Depression and the body pain was assessed by the Medical Outcome Survey (SF-36). Longer-term treatment response was measured using the Bodily Pain Index.

The key findings were that 141 (75%) of the subjects responded to combined treatment and the rest needed further augmentation treatment with drugs. No direct relationship was found between levels of body pain and suicidal ideation. However, the fact that combined treatment could produce such a robust outcome even for patients with substantial body pain was very positive. The authors concluded that coexisting pain and medical illness in older adult outpatients with depression need not be barriers to satisfactory treatment response. However, they cautioned that the complex nature of the relationship between body pain and depression required further study.

The second was a clinical article that explained the significance of the interpersonal model for understanding somatizing behavior (Stuart and Noyes, 2006). Somatizing behavior, as per this model, is deemed to be a form of interpersonal communication driven by insecure attachments. The authors reported on their experience of using IPT on somatizing patients with strategies that included an emphasis on therapeutic alliance and aimed for improvement in interpersonal functioning rather than in the alleviation of physical symptoms.

The success of IPT in treating depressed individuals with significant psychosocial problems has been considerable. Mufson et al. (2006) clearly showed the efficacy of IPT in treating adolescent depression. In a controlled study, 48 clinically depressed adolescents between the ages of 12 and 18 were randomly assigned to IPT or clinical monitoring. Treatment was spread over a 12-week period. Their progress was monitored biweekly by a "blind" independent evaluator to assess their social functioning, problem-solving skills, and symptoms. A total of 75% of IPT recipients as compared with 46% in the control group met the recovery criterion for depression at week 12. However, there were a number of limitations in the study such as small sample size, substantial attrition from the control group, and the use of self-report measures of social functioning, which made their findings somewhat preliminary. Nevertheless, the findings of this study justify the use of IPT for adolescent patients.

Similarly, IPT has been shown to be effective in treating adult patients with myocardial infarction (Stuart and Cole, 1996). One of the lessons of this particular study was the necessity of modifying some of the tenets of IPT to suit the specific circumstances of postmyocardial patients. This is a case report of a successfully treated postmyocardial patient using a modified IPT. He manifested symptoms of depression not uncommon in postmyocardial patients. After 12 sessions, his score on Beck Depression Inventory (BDI) fell from a high of 28 (firmly in the clinical range) to 2 (nondepressed). He showed a similar decline on the Hamilton Rating Scale for Depression. This man eventually returned to work, and was free of symptoms commonly associated with depression.

HIV-positive patients have also responded positively to IPT (Markowitz et al., 1998). This was an RCT comparing CBT, IPT, and supportive psychotherapy with imipramine for HIV-positive patients with depression. A total of 101 subjects were randomized to 16 weeks of treatment. Inclusion criteria included a score of 15 or more on the Hamilton Rating Scale for Depression, clinical judgment of depression, and poor physical health requiring outpatient attendance. Subjects randomized to IPT and supportive psychotherapy with imipramine showed significantly greater improvement than the other two treatment groups. The authors concluded that IPT was especially effective in treating HIV-positive patients who had also experienced recent negative life events. IPT directly connected life events that enabled the patients to mourn upheavals while pragmatically and optimistically encouraging them to find new goals (Markowitz et al., 1998).

The application of IPT to treat a wide range of disorders such as bulimia nervosa (Fairburn et al., 1995), social phobia (Lipstiz et al., 1999), and obesity associated with binge-eating disorder (Wilfley et al., 2002) has met with considerable success. Again it is noteworthy that modifications were made to accommodate specific problems related to specific situations. For instance, in the treatment of bulimia the IPT protocol differed from the protocol for depression in two significant ways. First, the psychoeducational component that focused on the disorder itself was eliminated. Role playing and problem solving were taken out of the protocol as well. The point is that IPT lends itself to modification without losing its key tenets or compromising its effectiveness.

Swanston et al. (2000) following their review of psychotherapy outcome literature for treating young people with chronic medical conditions were optimistic about a whole range of interventions, such as supportive psychotherapy, telephone support, and home-based support, that seemed effective in enhancing their psychological adjustment. However, the authors made the critical observation that a solid scientific foundation for developing interventions in this critical area was wanting.

It has to be acknowledged that IPT has so far seen limited application to the adolescent population. Although Mufson et al. (2006) showed its effectiveness in the treatment of adolescent depression, this study had a number of serious limitations. It is also interesting that the subjects in the bulimia study were mostly adults or older adolescents. Therefore, our choice of IPT for treating Lisa was not to any significant degree based on its effectiveness with adolescents. Rather, the principles upon which IPT are predicated seemed highly relevant. We discuss these issues in the following section.

Tsi-Wai Chan's article (2005) has some direct relevance to Lisa's case as he considers IPT for depressed adolescents with chronic medical problems. Grief and loss due to chronic health problems and interpersonal role disputes with parents and peers as a consequence of illness and issues of role transition that can be seriously disrupted by chronic illness are all carefully analyzed in this article. The author noted that many adolescents confronted with the death of a parent showed marked withdrawal from relationships because they avoided intimacy or became preoccupied with fantasies of lost relationships. Critically, mourning often extended over a long period owing to the developmental tasks that confronted adolescents, sanctions against emotional expression, and the difficulties others had in perceiving their needs. In Lisa's case, it was not the loss of a parent but another kind of loss that produced similar reactions. She was acutely aware of falling behind her peers and of her overreliance on her mother, and as emerged in the course of therapy, she was reluctant to express her feelings of loss to anyone. Hence, she drew dark pictures depicting herself as a prisoner in a room without a door.

Tsi-Wai Chan (2005) offers a careful rationale for the use of IPT for adolescents with chronic illness. He also notes some of the common problems in engaging adolescents in any form of psychotherapy, and the fact that it takes some extra effort to establish a therapeutic relationship based on trust with an adolescent patient. Involvement of the parents in therapy is also recognized as a critical factor for the IPT to succeed. It is noteworthy that Lisa's mother, in particular, played a major role in Lisa's recovery.

Tsi-Wai Chan (2005) recognized the need to modify IPT to suit the needs of adolescent patients suffering from chronic illness. First is the necessity of parental involvement as an integral component of IPT. Second is the need for the therapist to collaborate with other healthcare providers to ensure that treatment goals are shared and supported. Although the author did not include the school system in this collaborative effort, this is another component that should be incorporated in the overall management of the child. Finally, the frequency and duration should be adapted to the specific circumstances of the patient. Both may have to be modified to the specific needs of the child. In our treatment of Lisa the prescribed length of therapy exceeded beyond the IPT recommended sessions by virtue of the severity of her emotional dislocation and attending health problems. Lisa continued to be seen beyond the active phase of therapy. Several authors have noted the necessity of maintenance IPT (in Lisa's case it was more in the way of regular review) for patients with recurring depression that can reduce relapse rates and prolong periods between depressive episodes (Frank et al., 1990; Reynolds et al., 1999).

Summary

At this point we return to Lisa's story to understand how IPT, with significant modification but without compromising its essential elements, proved to be highly successful in treating Lisa, and in significant measure restoring her normal adolescent struggles and preoccupations. When the four critical areas of concern for IPT, namely, grief, interpersonal role disputes, role transition, and interpersonal deficits, are applied to Lisa, they barely need further elaboration.

Grief was at the very heart of this case. For an emerging adolescent the loss of a uterus and the insult inflicted on self-image was complicated by the parents' religious interpretation of this event as being due to divine retribution, which created an optimum condition for Lisa's mental state. Besides, during her prolonged hospitalization, she came face to face with the death of a number of children she had known. She seemed mature beyond her years, yet her personal development was compromised.

She could not fit into the adolescent world of her peers and school. All these factors profoundly affected all other aspects of her relationships. For example, Lisa experienced enormous difficulties in the domain of interpersonal functioning. She was caught in a classical conflict of wanting and not wanting to be a part of her peer group. She was virtually friendless. She saw her peers as superficial, preoccupied with their clothes and boys. Yet, as the therapy progressed she gradually did integrate with her peer group showing ever-increasing interest in her appearance and in a particular boy.

IPT provided a method of intervention that seemed to be designed for Lisa's needs. Yet, it must be acknowledged that significant modification had to be made in terms of both the number of sessions and frequency. These are important issues when working with medically ill populations as health problems often need urgent attention and the fluctuation in the health status sometimes compromises the weekly sessions. However, what is being contented here is that IPT has sufficient flexibility to be adjusted to the peculiar needs of a patient. Another point of note in relation to Lisa is that even after IPT, she was kept under review for a long time. Altogether, Lisa's treatment lasted about a year and she emerged from this experience as a reasonably well-functioning adolescent.

At this point we turn our attention to the case of Clara, a middle-age married woman, with a very complicated medical history. Below is a summary of her problems and her response to IPT. Clara was referred to a pain clinic with complaints of burning bilateral foot and leg pain. Some 12 years earlier she had a stroke, which left her with compromised memory. She also had pregnancy-induced hypertension for both children as well as gestational diabetes. Past surgeries included tonsellectomy, appendectomy, ovarian cystectomy, knee surgery, cholecystectomy, and a breast reduction, which revealed precancerous growths. She was also facing a significant weight problem. In addition, she had hypothyroidism, pernicious anemia, and diet-controlled diabetes.

Clara's psychosocial history was equally complex. She grew up in a small town in the United Kingdom, her parents emigrating to Canada when she was a small child. She was a sickly child missing a great deal of school. Her home environment was far from stable. Eventually, her parents separated when Clara was 14. Clara revealed that she was sexually abused by her grandfather from the age of $4^1/_2$ to 9. Her developmental years were hugely disruptive because of health problems, abuse, and a very acrimonious family environment. She was a very poor scholar. Through all of this her mother subjected Clara to ongoing emotional abuse that continued well after she left home. This abuse took the form of constant criticism of Clara, her lack of intelligence, and the fact that she had been nothing but trouble ever since she was born.

Clara left home at the earliest opportunity and had the good fortune of meeting and marrying a man who provided her with the kind of affection and security that she never experienced as a child. There are two children: a son aged 21 and a daughter aged 18. The children have done well in school, and despite Clara's multiple health problems, this family showed a high level of cohesion. Yet, Clara was guilt-ridden about her inability to do all she wanted to do with the children. The same feelings also extended to her husband. She felt that she had been a burden. As for her sexual abuse, she had therapy and had come to terms with her past, but every now and again she invoked her past to justify her current dilemmas.

Clara at the point of her inception at the pain clinic was very upset and sad. Her social life was limited and her family life was problematic because she had to depend on her husband and daughter for so much. Their son was living on his own, but still very involved with the family. She was particularly distressed about her daughter because so much was taken away from her because of Clara's health problems. On days that she felt better, she generally tended to be overactive and paid a price in terms of more pain. Control or lack thereof was a major issue for her. She was reluctant at all times to ask for help. These issues defined her relationships and contributed significantly to her interpersonal conflicts.

As for her psychological state she did not appear to be unduly sad. However, on probing she revealed suicidal thoughts in the way that she wished she was dead. She did not actively entertain thoughts of killing herself, but did not see the purpose of living. She constantly fell back on her childhood to explain her lack of self-confidence and pervasive guilt. She was found to be moderately depressed. Therapy was offered, which she readily accepted. She had found therapy to be helpful in the past.

Our rationale for selecting IPT for Clara was based on what we perceived to be long-term moderate depression that had remained impervious to drugs. Our impression was that her depression was deeply rooted in her negative past and hugely compromised health and a profound sense of sadness and hopelessness, which she sometimes managed to conceal. The fact that she was in a very supportive long-term relationship with her husband and had raised two very intelligent and able and caring children did not seem to counteract her deep feelings of failure.

IPT, with its focus on interpersonal issues that often tend to get distorted by depression, seemed appropriate for Clara. However, at the very center of her problems was grief about her lost childhood, persistent health problems, an emotionally abusive mother, and indeed sexual abuse. These factors had led to major problems in all her relationships, particularly with her children and husband. The focus of therapy was to address the issues of grief related more directly to her ongoing health problems and its impact on her relationships. Her role as a mother, despite her chronic and multiple health problems, had to be seen from the perspective of the children. They were frustrated with her because they could not always relate to her self-deprecation. They wanted her to be more open with her feelings. Strategies included communication analysis, which enabled the patient to communicate more effectively with her family members and understand and manage her feelings, very targeted questioning, and the exploration and clarification of the critical aspects of her current situation. The two areas of focus were grief and perceived role deficits. These deficits were mainly the products of her health problems, and clarification and education around these issues remained some of the key ingredients of this therapy.

She has been in therapy for 9 weeks before she acknowledged that her thoughts about not wanting to live had virtually disappeared. She was beginning to appreciate that her children did not see her as an uncaring and demanding mother. She felt a little freer in asking them for help, albeit, reluctantly. She was encouraged to have these conversations. She was more successful in opening up to her daughter than to either her husband or her son. In sum, she showed considerable improvement with therapy.

Again, her therapy had to be modified as she missed a number of sessions because of pain, but she remained committed. At the time of writing, she remains engaged in therapy. Her husband reported seeing a major change in her attitude for the better. She was more open with her feelings and far less self-critical and, most importantly, little less demanding on herself.

Accounts of IPT to treat medically complex cases like Clara's are hard to come by. We report one such case of a 60-year-old female patient with a complex medical and psychiatric history (Kaur, 2005). She had a history of alcohol dependence that began in her early twenties. She also had untreated posttraumatic stress disorder from childhood sexual and physical abuse and breast cancer. She still had flashbacks and nightmares and engaged in avoidance behaviors. Therefore, a combination of psychotherapy and medications was determined to be the most helpful treatment.

She was admitted to an extended care service, where she could be monitored. She began attending an intensive daycare program for her addictions. Her mirtazipine was discontinued because of her ongoing neutropenia. She was started on citalopram. She also received IPT once a week and was referred to a breast cancer support group. An important part of ongoing treatment has involved processing her shame and guilt related to her sexual traumas and dysfunctional relationship with her mother. Discussions on issues of death and dying were also useful. The report stated that she was continuing to do well.

There are some striking similarities between this case and Clara's. Child abuse and a very problematic relationship with her mother are the most obvious. They also shared serious health problems. Clara was not confronted with life and death issues, but she also encountered very serious health problems including cerebral vascular accidents (CVAs). Both these patients seem to be responding well to IPT and to medical treatment, which in Clara's case is mainly a complex regimen of analgesics. At least at the clinical level the application of IPT to patients with complex medical and relationship issues holds much promise.

Clara, a very challenging patient, with a complex medical history engaged in IPT with ease. She showed rapid progress and provided early evidence of overcoming issues that had remained unsolved. The quality of her relationships improved all around. Her mood was much better and she was far less self-deprecating. She was enthusiastic about her homework and applied herself diligently to therapy. Our expectation is that Clara will continue to gain from IPT.

Conclusion

Despite the very limited application of IPT in treating chronic pain patients, we have attempted to show its effectiveness in treating two very diverse cases representing very different types of problems. The truth is that social dislocation in the chronic pain population is of an epidemic proportion (Roy, 2001). Depression or at least depressive symptoms are commonly present. The social context in which these disruptions occur is self-evident. We chose two very different cases to show that with some modification (in Lisa's case), the choice of IPT made both common and clinical sense. In Clara's case, we were able to more or less adhere to the process outlined earlier. Her therapy continues.

IPT has proven an effective form of psychotherapy in treating depression. It would also seem that IPT lends itself to modification to conform to the specific needs of a patient. As could be seen from the review, although IPT is primarily a short-term therapy, there is considerable flexibility with regard to the actual number of sessions. There is also flexibility with the four elements of IPT in terms of which ones may or may not be pertinent to a particular situation. The fact that IPT is manualized is not in itself a restricting factor. Evidence of the success of IPT is impressive. RCTs have shown over and over again its power to treat depression. The literature on IPT has grown exponentially over the last decade or so. Even a cursory search on this topic can yield more than 200 articles and numerous books and manuals. The evidence of its success is less powerful with medically ill patients including patients with chronic pain, and only well-designed outcome studies can determine its true effectiveness.

References

deMello, M., deJusus, M., Mari, J., et al. (2005) A systemic review of research findings on the efficacy of interpersonal psychotherapy for depressive disorders. Eur. Arch. Psychiatry Neurosci., 255: 75–82.

Eccleston, C., Morley, S., Williams, A., et al. (2002) Systematic review of randomized control trials of psychological therapy for chronic pain in children and adolescents, with a subset meta-analysis of pain relief. Pain, 99: 157–165.

Elkin, I., Shea, M., Watkins, J., et al. (1989) National Institute of Mental Health Treatment of Depression Collaborative Research Program: general effectiveness of treatments. Arch. Gen. Psychiatry, 46: 971–982.

Fairburn, C., Norman, P., Welch, S., et al. (1995) A prospective study of outcome in bulimia nervosa and the effects of three psychological treatments. Arch. Gen. Psychiatry, 52: 304–312.

Frank, E., Kupfer, D., Perel, J., et al. (1990) Three year outcome maintenance therapies in recurrent depression. Arch. Gen. Psychiatry, 47: 1093–1099.

Karp, J., Weiner, D., Seligman, K., et al. (2005) Body pain and treatment response in late-life depression. Am. J. Geriatr. Psychiatry, 13: 188–194.

Kaur, N. (2005) A 60 year old woman with multiple psychiatric and medical conditions. Psychiatr. Ann., 35: 111–115.

Klein, D. and Ross, D. (1993) Reanalysis of the National Institute of Mental Health Treatment of Depression Collaborative Research Program: General effectiveness report. Neuropsychopharmacology, 8: 241.

Kotova, E. (2005) A meta-analysis of interpersonal psychotherapy. Dissertation Abstracts. Section B: The Science and Engineering, 66(5-B).

Leibing, E., Rabung, S., and Leichsenring, F. (2005) About the efficacy of short-term psychodynamic psychotherapy in the treatment of psychic disorders. Forum Psychoanalyse klinische Theorie Praxis, 21: 371–379.

Lipstiz, J., Markowitz, J., Cherry, S., and Friaer, A. (1999) Open trial for interpersonal therapy for the treatment of social phobia. Am. J. Psychiatry, 156: 1814–1816.

Markowitz, J., Kocsis, J., Fishman, B., et al. (1998) Treatment of depressive symptoms in human immunodeficiency virus-positive patients. Arch. Gen. Psychiatry, 55: 452–457.

Merlijn, V., Hunfeld, J., van der Wouden, J., et al. (2006) Factors related to the quality of life in adolescents with chronic pain. Clin. J. Pain, 22: 306–315.

Merlijn, V., Hunfeld, J., van der Wouden, J., et al. (2003) Psychosocial factors associated with chronic pain in adolescents. Pain, 101: 33–43.

Mufson, L. Dorta, K.P., Moreau, D., and Weissman, M.M. (2004) Interpersonal Psychotherapy for Depressed Adolescents, 2nd edn. New York, Guilford Press.

Mufson, L., Weissman, M., Moreau, D., and Garfinkel, R. (2006) Efficacy of interpersonal psychotherapy for depressed adolescents. Arch. Gen. Psychiatry, 56: 573–579.

Ravitz, P. (2004) Evidence-based psychotherapies—The interpersonal fulcrum: interpersonal therapy to treatment of depression. Canadian Psychiatric Association Bulletin.

Reynolds, C., Frank, E., Perel, J., et al. (1999) Nortriptyline and interpersonal psychotherapy as maintenance therapies for recurrent major depression: a randomized controlled trial in patients older than 59 years. JAMA, 281: 39–45.

Roy, R. (2001) Social Relations and Chronic Pain. New York, Kluwer Academic/Plenum Publishers.

Roy, R. (2004) Chronic Pain, Loss and Suffering. Toronto, University of Toronto Press.

Salsman, N. (2006) Interpersonal change as an outcome of time-limited interpersonal psychotherapy. Dissertation Abstracts International. Section B: The Sciences and Engineering, 69(9B).

Stuart, S. and Cole, V. (1996) Treatment of depression following myocardial infarction with interpersonal psychotherapy. Ann. Clin. Psychiatry, 8: 203–206.

Stuart, S. and Robertson, M. (2003) Interpersonal Psychotherapy: A Clinician's Guide. London, Arnold.

Stuart, S. and Noyes, R. (2006) Interpersonal psychotherapy for somatizing patients. Psychother. Psychosom., 75: 209–219.

Swanston, H., Williams, K., and Nunn, K. (2000) The psychological adjustment of children with chronic conditions. In: Kosky, R., O'Hanlon, A., Martin, G., and Davis, C. (Series Eds.)

Clinical Approaches to Early Intervention in Child and Adolescent Mental Health, Vol. 4. Adelaide, Australia, Australian Early Intervention Network for Mental Health in Young People.

Tsi-Wai Chan, R. (2005) Interpersonal psychotherapy as a treatment model for depressed adolescents with chronic medical problems. Clin. Child Psychol. Psychiatry, 10: 88–101.

Weissman, M., Markowitz, J., and Klerman, G. (2000) Comprehensive Guide to Interpersonal Psychotherapy. New York, Basic Books.

Weel, S., Merlijn, V., Passchier, J., et al. (2005) Development and psychometric properties on pain-related problem list for adolescents. Patient Educ. Couns., 58: 209–215.

Wilfley, D., Welch, R., Stein, R., et al. (2002) A randomized comparison of group cognitive-behavioral therapy and group interpersonal psychotherapy for the treatment of overweight individuals with binge-eating disorder. Arch. Gen. Psychiatry, 59: 317–320.

Chapter 6
Grief Therapy

Although grief associated with loss of roles and functions is commonly observed in the chronically ill population, including chronic pain sufferers, the literature dealing with this critical topic is conspicuously scarce (Roy, 2004). There is widespread acknowledgment that chronic pain has far-reaching consequences for those suffering from it. They can experience social dislocation of some magnitude (Roy, 2001). These may include loss of employment, and significant loss of social and family roles, activities, and mobility, among others (Roy, 2007). What is noteworthy, as our literature review will show, is that psychosocial intervention to help these patients deal with these multiple losses has gone virtually unnoticed. Although the literature on grief therapy associated with death is rich, such a claim cannot be made for losses related to chronic illness.

We have chosen three very different cases to illustrate the dilemma. Our first case fits into the more traditional understanding of grief, involving multiple deaths leading to pathological grief. The second case involves a young woman affected by rheumatoid arthritis, with very serious consequences on her life in general and on her self-esteem in particular. We present a vignette of the third case to demonstrate the difficult path our patients have to travel to reach some level of acceptance of their pain and associated disabilities, and how they somehow fail to attain that objective.

Tina, a woman in her early fifties with a complicated history of abdominal pain related to pyoderma and multiple surgeries, was referred to the pain clinic for pain management. Routine psychosocial investigation revealed some alarming facts. Some 18 months earlier, her husband died unexpectedly and in a most unusual manner. He had mistakenly taken the wrong medicine (his wife's) and that caused his death. There was an inquest and indeed a police investigation and the death was ruled accidental. Soon after, her mother died of natural causes. Six months after her death, her elderly father committed suicide.

She had been living the life of a recluse. Her relationship with her three grown-up children was tenuous at best. She acknowledged that she always put on a great front in the presence of her children. Otherwise, she was sad all the time, cried frequently, and could not come to terms with the fact her own medication caused her husband's death. She had been showing all the elements of abnormal grief; the main characteristic was depression, not an uncommon reaction in the face of two traumatic deaths. She was totally guilt-ridden. She was difficult to engage in therapy.

R. Roy, *Psychosocial Interventions for Chronic Pain*,
DOI: 10.1007/978-0-387-76296-8_6 © Springer Science+Business Media, LLC 2008

Initially, we adopted a cognitive behavioral approach in the hope that she would be able to see the reality as it was (thorough clarification and re-attribution) and accept the reality of her husband's death. We were only nominally successful. She was also being treated with anti-depressants by her family physician, but without any obvious benefit.

It took a great deal of persuasion for her to agree to a psychiatric evaluation. The psychiatrist diagnosed her as undergoing a "major depressive episode as well as a complicated grief reaction." He revised her medication and commenced aggressive treatment for her depression and recommended ongoing grief therapy. All this took place about a year since her inception into the pain clinic. We also changed our therapeutic approach by adopting a more conventional grief therapy approach, the key element of which was to enable the patient to engage in catharsis, and slowly begin the process of acceptance that her husband's death was accidental and that she had no control over her father's suicide, and begin the process of re-defining herself and her relationships, and begin the complicated process of finding meaning in these losses. At the time of writing, she has been with us for nearly 2 years, and finally showing signs of recovery and rejuvenation. It is also noteworthy that through all her ordeal, her pain which brought her to the pain clinic in the first place, receded into the background. In fact, she rarely complained about her pain.

Our next patient, June, in her early twenties, represents many chronic pain sufferers who encounter multitude of changes in their roles and activities. She was diagnosed with rheumatoid arthritis in her late teens. The disease remained under control for some years. She finished high school and started working as a veterinary assistant. She loved animals and loved her job. A year before her disease became active, she married a man she had known for several years. She resisted visiting her physician for several months although her disease had entered an active phase. In the meantime, her job was becoming increasingly burdensome. Soon after, she was dismissed unceremoniously for poor performance. This job loss was a profound shock to June, and the very first concrete evidence that she was having difficulty in coping with many of her activities. Her defenses were coming apart.

After her job loss, June went through, what can only be described as, a personality change. She avoided any human interaction and cried frequently, and paradoxically engaged in heavy chores that were not essential. It was in this state that she was sent by her family physician to a pain clinic for psychosocial assessment and therapy. June had coped with her illness mainly through denial and still tried to do so at great personal cost. In summary, she lost her job, was confronted with declining physical abilities and loss of meaningful social roles. Her spousal role was also severely compromised.

June remained in therapy for approximately 18 months. The therapeutic process was based in the loss-restoration approach. Loss orientation is focused on the losses experienced. June had encountered many such significant losses. During the first phase of therapy she was in a state of acute grief and cried through most of the sessions, saying very little. For the next several months, she showed two distinct sources of preoccupation. First was her monthly blood test that revealed the level of disease activity, and second was her sense of profound humiliation associated with her dismissal from her job. Gradually, June's range of focus expanded to include the whole gamut of losses that had robbed her of any sense of who she was and her purpose in life. During this entire phase, June remained very negative and sad, and this was when her self-esteem was at its lowest.

The restoration phase began almost imperceptibly. One of the early signs of it was her ability on "good" days to engage in activities that seemed commensurate with her ability rather than overdoing it as in the past. This was an indication of her recognition of the limits imposed on her by the disease. At this point, June also decided to inform herself about her disease. She was beginning to have some control over her situation. Her crying had become very rare. She began to take an interest in her husband's plumbing business. She began to talk about her deep love of horses and of her experience at the animal hospital. One day she made an unexpected announcement to the therapist that she had been volunteering at a local day care for a couple of hours a day and was having a very good time interacting with the children. These were the early signs of reintegration and finding alternative sources for enjoyment and gratification which came about through her search for meaningful activities.

The long process of redefining her identity had commenced. She started taking an interest in her husband's business and gradually became his business manager. She enrolled in a computer program to learn accounting. By the time of the termination of therapy, she had achieved two essential goals. First, she came to terms with living with a chronic illness with all its vagaries, and second, she found meaningful activities, and thus began the process of redefining her identity. Her self-esteem was restored to a very significant degree. Two other facts contributed to her recovery: first, a remarkably understanding husband, and second, her exceptionally supportive parents. At the point of discharge, she was advised, if necessary, to contact the clinic. That was more than 6 years ago.

Our third patient, John, a man in his sixties presented with a history of severe neuropathic foot pain. He harbored a great deal of resentment from the very beginning of his problem some 7 years ago. Soon after the onset of his pain, he was forced to give up his job that involved a great deal of travel. His attitude was one of anger and resentment and sometimes deep sadness. He often contemplated suicide. Seven years on, his condition has remained refractory to treatment(s). Only opioid medication provides him with relief. His resentment has grown, as has his anger. He responded partially to CBT, but failed to benefit from relaxation training. His suicidal thoughts come and go. Antidepressant medications have not produced any significant effect on this man. He remains in supportive therapy.

Grief Therapy and Outcome: A Literature Review

Grief associated with chronic illness is a grossly underresearched area. Much of what we can claim about its efficacy for treating the chronic pain population is, at best, indirect. On the other hand, the fact that the process of grieving, regardless of the nature of loss, tends to be somewhat similar cannot be denied. This fact was amply demonstrated by the work of Colin Murray Parkes (1973), Parkes and Weiss (1983), who demonstrated the similarity in the grieving process between loss of a spouse and loss of limb. Much of the literature on grief therapy concerns death and dying. Coming to terms with one's own impending death, and working through the process of bereavement after the death of a loved one are the central aspects of published material on grief therapy. Types of grief therapy are wide ranging—from catharsis to family oriented to cognitive behavioral to egooriented to all varieties of group therapy (Roy, 2004). As our review will show, grief therapy falls into three broad categories: (1) family based, (2) group based, and (3) individually based. We shall review the most recent literature on outcome in all three types of interventions. Finally, we shall report on the literature on grief therapy to treat grief associated with chronic illness including chronic pain. Many authors are claiming that our understanding of the grieving process is undergoing a revolution—from the psychodynamic base to a more psychosocial orientation. The phase-task orientation, upon which so much of the grieving process is predicated, is under scrutiny. Neimeyer (1999) noted some of the new elements:

1. Scepticism regarding the predictability of the pathways leading from a state of disequilibrium to acceptance;
2. A shift away from letting-go of the deceased (or any other loss) to maintain symbolic bonds with the lost "object";
3. Attention to the meaning-making process that mourning entails, as well as to the specific symptomatic and emotional consequences of that loss (potential for abnormal grief);
4. Attention to the altered identity of the bereaved (or a person who may have lost a limb or a job through illness);
5. Focus on post-loss growth and integration of the lessons learned in connection with the loss; and
6. Shifting the focus from the individual to the whole family.

Literature Review

We focus on outcome studies that involve, minimally, a control group although they may fail to meet the rigors of a randomized control trial.

Meta-analyses and Other Reviews of Grief Therapy Outcome Literature

Allambaugh and Hoyt (1999) used meta-analysis to address the question of the efficacy of grief therapy. Their analysis was based on 35 studies. The studies were included based on the following criteria: They examined the efficacy of any type of grief therapy, had a comparison group for the treated group or compared pre-treatment post-treatment scores for treated participants, and reported sufficient data to facilitate statistical analysis.

The findings were complex. Modality of intervention indicated a trend for group treatment to be less effective than individual interventions. Authors acknowledged that this finding ran counter to the finding of comparability in the general psychotherapy outcome literature. We shall revisit this question in our review of group therapy.

In terms of client characteristics, level of client risk for complicated grief was unrelated to outcome. Low-risk clients derived roughly the same level of benefit as did high-risk clients. However, the definition of "high-risk clients" differed from study to study. This may, in part, explain lack of significance. Length of treatment produced some equivocal evidence of a linear relation between treatment length and efficacy. However, much of the treatment in these studies tended to be brief.

Outcome was in the predictable direction. Clients in the no-treatment control groups showed little improvement, possibly because of the relatively long delay between loss and treatment in most studies (27 months). Moderators of treatment efficacy included time since loss and relationship to the deceased. A small number of studies involving self-selected clients produced relatively large effect size, whereas the majority of studies involving clients recruited by the investigators produced effect size in the small-to-moderate range. Self-selection combined with individual therapy emerged as the best predictors for successful outcome. However, one major limitation of this review was that it included a number of uncontrolled one-group studies that could have inflated estimates of efficacy of the therapies included.

The review discussed next confirms some of the key findings and contradicts others of the preceding report (Fortner, 2000). This review is based on 23 controlled experiments on grief counseling and therapy. Overall results showed a relatively small positive effect. However, an astounding 37% of participants in therapy were worse off at post-test, and they were described as treatment-induced deterioration. Complicated grief responded most effectively to intervention. This was confirmed by a small number of studies involving complicated grief. This review came to a tentative conclusion that grief counseling and therapy was likely to be the most effective for individuals experiencing complicated grief, which usually manifested as prolonged grief, anxiety, and mood disorders. The author urged more focused research with this population.

Our final review in this section is a report of published randomized controlled outcome studies of grief counseling and therapy (Neimeyer, 2000). This review confirmed Fortner's (2000) finding that grief therapy was typically ineffective and even deleterious at least for persons experiencing normal grief, and likely to be more effective with those who have been traumatically bereaved.

Neimeyer (2000) noted that despite the huge proliferation of literature on grief therapy, only RCTs yielded a clear verdict on the efficacy of this therapy. They found 23 papers published between 1975 and 1998 meeting their rigorous criteria. Some 1600 participants in these studies had lost a spouse, children, or other family members and received some form of psychosocial intervention such as psychotherapy, counseling, or group therapy. Professionals provided therapy in 19 of these studies.

Most of these studies measured outcome on common measures of health, such as anxiety, depression, or psychiatric distress, and only a few tried to measure grief per se. Although in general terms, subjects clearly benefited from therapy compared to the non-treatment groups, the average participant in grief therapy was better-off of bereaved persons who received no treatment at all by only 55%.

More telling was the finding that nearly 38% of recipients of grief therapy theoretically would have been better-off if assigned to no-treatment groups. The conclusion was that "not only is the tangible benefit of grief therapy small, but its risk of producing iatrogenic worsening of problems is unacceptably high" (Neimeyer, 2000, p. 545).

Summary

Conclusions to be drawn from these three reviews are complex. Not only is grief therapy not helpful, it may even be harmful when applied to persons going through normal grieving. However, its potential as a means of treating abnormal or pathological grief is significant. Can any inferences be drawn from these reviews about the applicability of grief therapy in treating chronic pain sufferers who may be experiencing grief to one degree or another due to many reversals of fortune in their lives? It would seem, even on the basis of two of our case illustrations, that severity of grief may be just as relevant as it is to death-related grief. The fact derived from these reviews is that grieving is a common, predictable, and even desirable response to loss, and a vast majority of people emerge from this experience without having to resort to expert intervention.

In the section that follows, we report on a number of studies involving groups and individuals. The final section will review the literature on chronic illness and grief therapy. Our literature search shows that family approach is widely adopted to treat bereaved families. However, outcome studies to test its efficacy are conspicuous by their absence. One report on family-focused grief therapy during palliative care tried to evaluate treatment integrity of Family Focused Grief Therapy (FFGT) (Chan et al., 2004). This was a randomized controlled study, but the purpose of the study was not so much as to test the efficacy of FFGT, but rather the degree to which the therapists adhered to the core elements of the model. Authors of this study demonstrated the consistency with which a brief, family-focused model of family therapy designed specifically to support high-risk families during palliative care and subsequent bereavement was used by therapists. Efficacy of family therapy for grief remains unknown. Although the clinical literature on that topic is rich and varied and indeed very considerable, this gap in the literature is hard to explain.

Group Therapy

Research into the efficacy of group therapy for bereavement has yielded positive results. Much of this research in recent years has been conducted by Ogrodniczuk and his associates, which includes level of alliance and alliance over sessions and outcome (Piper et al., 2005), negative effects of alexithymia on outcome (Ogrodniczuk et al., 2005), differences in responses to grief therapy between men and women (Ogrodniczuk et al., 2004), quality of object relation and outcome (Piper et al., 2003), personality variables and outcome (Ogrodniczuk et al., 2003), social support as predictor of outcome (Ogrodniczuk et al., 2002a), influence of affect and work on outcome (Piper et al., 2002), and affect and outcome (McCullum et al., 1993). Sikkema et al. (2004) reported on an RCT of group intervention for HIV-positive men and women coping with AIDS-related deaths and bereavement. We present a brief selected review of this literature.

Sikkema and associates reported on the efficacy of cognitive behavioral group therapy in treating grief in a group of HIV-positive subjects. The sample consisted of 150 men and 85 women ranging in age between 21 years and 60 years. They represented several ethnic groups, the predominant one being African American. Fifty-two and 33 women were randomly assigned to intervention and comparison groups, as were 87 and 63 men respectively. Psychiatric screening revealed that all study participants had a lifetime history of psychiatric diagnosis, and psychiatric morbidity was common. Substance abuse and mood and anxiety disorders and borderline personality disorders were the most common disorders. Four therapists provided all the treatment. They had extensive experience in group therapy methods. Steps were taken to ensure adherence to the protocol.

Experimental intervention comprised of 12 weekly sessions of cognitive behavioral and supportive group therapy of 90-minute duration each. The comparison condition consisted of approximated what the patients would normally receive. Services were provided by masters-level and doctoral-level therapists.

Results showed that women and heterosexual men receiving the experimental intervention improved in grief-related distress significantly more than women and heterosexual men in the comparison condition. However, subjects in both treatment groups showed significant improvement, indicating that the treatment condition to which they were assigned did not have a significant impact on the outcome. Women in the experimental intervention group demonstrated the greatest positive change. Men, however, showed improvement in both treatment conditions. Further analysis of the grief and depression measures revealed significant gender differences—women receiving the intervention improving the most and men improving whether they the received the intervention or not.

The authors concluded that despite the fact that overall improvement was modest and primarily gender-specific, they were consistent with previous findings. They offered three reasons for the modest overall improvement, which was mainly gender-specific. First, grief had a natural history and recovery generally occurred as a matter of course. Second, participants in the control group received a significant amount of support and therapy, which included 12 weeks of individual psychotherapy, and psychological and psychiatric help was available on demand. Third, repeated contact with all the participants in this study may have also contributed to overall improvement. They were appreciative of the focus on grief of this study, which was often not addressed in regular services they received.

As noted earlier, Ogrodniczuk and colleagues (2003) have examined the influence of many and diverse factors on the outcome of group therapy for complicated grief. One of the studies reported by Ogrodniczuk et al. (2004) confirmed the findings of the above study. They investigated differences in men's and women's responses to short-term group psychotherapy. These individuals were suffering from complicated grief due to death-related losses. Patients were assigned to two forms (interpretive and supportive) of brief group psychotherapy. Findings showed that women generally had a better outcome compared to men in both forms of interventions. Authors noted that men were less committed to their therapy groups, and more importantly, they were perceived by other group members to be less compatible than women. The fact that men received less benefit from group therapy appears to have some credence.

Another study by Ogrodniczuk and associates (2002b) examined the role of social support as a predictor to group therapy for complicated grief. Conducted among psychiatric outpatients, 107 subjects between the ages of 19 and 67, who received either interpretive or supportive group therapy, rated their perceptions of social support from family, friends, and a special person. For both groups, perceived social support from friends resulted in positive outcome. The reverse was true for social support from family members. Support from a special person was found to be favorable for improvement in grief symptomatology for patients in the interpretive group, but not so in the supportive group. The results, overall, highlighted a long-standing assertion about the value of social support. On the other hand, the findings about family support, which was not helpful, were somewhat counterintuitive as spousal support has long been established as a powerful moderator of stress.

The final study we report on the outcome of group therapy investigated the influence of cohesion and alliance on the outcome of a psychodynamically based group therapy program to treat complicated grief (McNeil, 2006). Subjects included 79 women and 20 men who were randomly assigned to either supportive or interpretive group therapy. Fourteen outcome measures were completed three times (pretherapy, post-therapy, and 6-month follow-up). For cohesion and alliance, strongest relationships were observed at the beginning and at the end stage of therapy. Improvement was noted in both groups. Patient-rated alliance proved to be a better predictor than cohesion. This study showed the importance of taking into account two critical aspects of therapy that might influence outcome.

Summary

Grief therapy has come under significant scrutiny over the past decade or so, and the efficacy of this method to treat complicated grief has been noted. Again, it is noteworthy that all the studies reviewed here involved complicated grief. The other point of note is that supportive group therapy was often as effective as interpretive group therapy. It would appear that the type of group therapy was of less importance than the fact that group process itself was of therapeutic value. The data is unequivocal in supporting the efficacy of group therapy for complicated grief. The quality of research can be described as good. The studies reported here had control groups and were methodologically acceptable.

Individual Interventions

Individual interventions consist of a plethora of psychotherapies that range from psychodynamic to Internet-based interventions. However, it is the cognitive behavioral therapy (CBT) to treat grief that has, perhaps, received the highest level of empirical support.

Malkinson (2001), in her wide-ranging review of the grief therapy literature, confirmed the efficacy of CBT as an effective form of intervention for complicated grief. She noted that many reviews of outcome studies that were cognitively oriented for treatment of post-traumatic stress disorder, depression, anxiety, and chronic or traumatic grief were found to be particularly effective. Cognitive therapies that focused on the belief system of an individual and consequent thoughts and behaviors were particularly well-suited for CBT.

Malkinson observed that many different types of interventions have emerged from CBT that can be effectively used for treating grief. One model that she singled out was Ellis-Hill's (1962, 1976, 1985, 1991) The Adversely-Beliefs Consequences (ABC) Model. This model is a useful tool to understand grief and bereavement. Applying this model to bereaved individuals helps separate normal response to grief from pathological. The rational emotive behavioral therapy (REBT), which emphasizes the centrality of the cognitive processes, helps to distinguish between healthy and unhealthy response to loss. The REBT utilizes a variety of interventions that are rooted in cognitively based interventions and Malkinson demonstrates its efficacy through case illustrations.

McCallum and colleagues (2003) compared four forms of short-term psychotherapy and relative strength of two patient characteristics (psychological mindedness and alexithymia, often characterized as the opposite sides of the same coin) as predictors of psychotherapy outcome. Patients suffering from complicated grief were randomly assigned to four therapy conditions. Data was obtained from two comparative trials of interpretive versus supportive therapy. The therapy approach (interpretive vs supportive) did not seem to affect the relationship between either predictor variable and outcome. However, there was significant direct relationship between psychological mindedness and favorable outcome, and between alexithymia and favorable outcome in both trials.

In both short-term group therapy and short-term individual therapy, alexithymia and psychological mindedness were associated with outcome. The investigators failed to find any evidence of an interaction between the patient variables and therapy approach and treatment outcome. Predictably, higher levels of psychological mindedness and lower level of alexithymia predicted positive outcome with all four forms of therapy. One major finding of clinical significance of this study was that patients most suited for psychotherapy, regardless of type, are those with high psychological mindedness and low alexithymia. Type of therapy did not influence outcome.

Finally, we report on an innovative approach to Internet-based CBT for complicated grief (Wagner et al., 2006). Symptoms of complicated grief included avoidance, intrusion, and failure to adapt. This randomized controlled trial investigated the efficacy of an Internet-based CBT therapy program for bereaved individuals suffering from complicated grief. This approach combined psychotherapy with new technology whereby therapists and patients communicated exclusively via e-mail. Treatment protocol consisted of 2 weekly writing assignments over a period of 5 weeks, with the therapist and the patients communicating via e-mail. Patients were initially educated about the psychoeducational underpinning of this method. Fifty-five patients were randomly assigned to either treatment group or waiting-list control condition. Twenty-six patients in the treatment group improved significantly relative to the subjects in the control group. Treatment resulted in significant reductions in the severity of the main symptoms and in depression and anxiety. The improvement was maintained at the 3-month follow-up. Authors were careful to point out that this type of intervention may not suit all patients. A full 41% of patients who requested this treatment did not meet the inclusion criteria. Nevertheless, this approach, involving low-cost and positive outcome, has much potential.

Summary

Individual-based CBT for complicated grief has been shown to have considerable efficacy. One of the studies we reviewed minimally showed that individual therapy was equally effective to group therapy. Our last report is notable for its ingenuity for marrying CBT with modern technology as an effective therapy for complicated grief. Individual supportive as well as interpretive psychotherapies have also been demonstrated as being efficacious in the treatment of complicated grief.

Grief Therapy for Chronic Pain and Illness Patients

Alonzo (2000), in a very thoughtful paper, made the following observation: "The pathophysiology that produces chronic disease does not begin at the symptom onset, and the psychological strategies to cope with a chronic illness, whether efficacious or maladaptive, also do not begin at symptom onset, but develop over the life course." This statement summarizes the underlying conceptual issues that surround the very idea of grief associated with chronic illness. This problem may also account for the paucity of research on grief therapy and chronic illness. Grief associated with chronic pain disorders, nevertheless, is to be commonly observed when looked for. Several studies have demonstrated a link between chronic diseases and depression, but as Bruce (1999) put it, by no means does every person with a physical disability become depressed or every person with depression become disabled. The level of disability combined with the psychological and social variables may account for resiliency in some individuals and lack of it in others.

Roy (2007) noted the high level of social dislocation that many patients with chronic pain experience. Not one aspect of their life remains unaffected by this affliction. Loss of employment, loss of valued roles, and social isolation combined with physical disability and pain create an optimum condition for depression and grief. Research has shown that physical limitation with all its implications is a major contributory factor in producing sadness, hopelessness, and even depression (Ellis-Hill and Horn, 2000; Vali and Walkup, 1998). The preceding review was unambiguous about the efficacy of psychotherapeutic interventions only with complicated grief. The question in relation to grief and chronic illness is the difficulty associated with identifying complicated grief, which often manifests as depression. Sadness and a sense of loss which are common accompaniments of chronic illness may take on clinical proportions any time during a patient's journey through the ups and downs of the medical condition. In the case of June, she experienced profound grief in the early stage of her illness. Many patients become increasingly despondent and even depressed to the point of being suicidal if they fail to achieve any significant improvement in their condition (Roy, 2004).

It is worth reiterating that there are qualitative differences between grief associated with a single trauma and grief that we witness in chronically ill patients. Often, there is an absence of trauma and even when a patient is forced to give up employment, such an event may not be altogether unanticipated. The process of grieving differs in another important respect. This is largely because chronic illness is on a continuum and has peaks and valleys, and the very idea of stages of grief from shock to resolution and acceptance is made redundant. The unpredictable nature of many chronic diseases complicates the grieving process.

Thompson and Kyle (2000) reported that chronically ill patients discover and adopt creative strategies for keeping on top of their lives in the face of serious odds. These strategies involve acceptance, establishing reachable goals, finding and creating control, and using humor. Control or more specifically the lack thereof over their activities is at the very core of the struggle of our patients.

We conducted a search of the Cochrane Reviews and failed to find any review on grief therapy per se. However, a number of reports related to psychological treatment for chronic illnesses were found. Close scrutiny of some of them revealed that grief-related issues manifesting as depression often prompted these studies. One illustration of that is the review of psychological therapies for persons with multiple sclerosis (MS) (Thomas et al., 2006). The authors noted that the impact of MS can be overwhelming, with the possibility of reduced physical function, with disruption in education (for young people), employment, sexual and family functioning, friendships, and activities of daily living (Thomas et al., 2006). Moreover, MS can have an impact on sense of self, especially if they can no longer perform valued activities. Most critically, the authors noted that anxiety and depression are often the products of difficulty in adjusting to and coping with the disease.

Sixteen relevant studies involving somewhat diverse group of studies in terms of therapeutic orientations, all RCTs, were included in this review. However, CBT, the authors cautiously concluded, could help patients with MS to deal with depression and in adjusting and coping with the disease. They concluded that although no definite conclusions could be reached based on this review, psychological interventions identified in this study could potentially help people with MS.

The two other Cochrane Reviews that had some bearing on the topic failed to establish efficacy of psychosocial interventions. Cystic fibrosis, which is a life-threatening disease, also has profound impact on the patients' abilities and relationships (Glasscoe and Quittner, 2006). The authors searched for randomized and quasi-randomized controlled trials. Findings were based on eight studies which ranged in scope from therapy to improve dietary intake to therapy to improve quality of life. The authors concluded that not enough of strong evidence emerged to clearly show whether these interventions improved outcome. The other review involved psychosocial interventions to combat depression in dialysis patients (Rabindranath et al., 2006). Authors concluded that data were not available to draw any conclusions about the efficacy of psychosocial interventions to treat depression in this population. The authors recommended that long-term studies were needed in this area. It must be emphasized that not one of these three studies made any direct reference to grief. Grief is more implicit in these studies, although the review involving MS patients was focused on issues related to loss, such as altered identity and loss of valued roles.

Amputation of a limb has received some clinical attention from the perspective of loss. These reports are anecdotal and they describe many new and novel approaches to grief therapy with this population. One report describes the process of grief therapy with a 13-year-old boy who had to undergo emergency surgery for the amputation of a leg (Judd, 2001). Nau (1997) described the benefits of letter writing; for example, writing to one's lost limb. This approach, according to the author, helped clients confront their loss and grieve in a meaningful way. Buttenshaw (1993) wrote at length the entire rehabilitation process including psychological interventions for amputees. Grief therapy for cancer-related losses has also received some clinical attention (Esplen et al., 2000; Fox and Rau, 2001; Hayashi, 1994; Swenson and Fuller, 1992). These reports describe a variety of interventions: family-focused, couple therapy, client-centered therapy, and so on.

We found two studies on chronic pain and grief therapy (Reed, 1999; Sagula and Rice, 2004), and we discuss them in some detail. Reed (1999) measured the efficacy of grief therapy for patients with chronic pain and depression in reducing or ameliorating these symptoms and enhancing their quality of life. It should be noted that depressive symptoms are ubiquitous in chronic pain sufferers. Among other measures, utilization of healthcare services, medication usage, and employment status were also measured. Sixty-one adult patients were randomly assigned to two groups. Both groups received standard treatment over a 5-month period, but the experimental group received the added grief therapy. Data were collected at three points over the study period. Results were unequivocal in showing the added power of grief therapy in reducing pain and depression, utilization of healthcare services, and reliance on psychotropic drugs. Grief therapy was effective in enhancing overall well-being, chances of returning to work, and/or entering vocational rehabilitation programs. However, utilization of health care and decrease in medication did not achieve statistical significance between the two groups, although there was a trend to in favor of the experimental group. This was the first study of this nature and established the possibility that combining standard treatment with grief therapy was more than likely to produce improved outcome.

Our final report investigated the effectiveness of mindfulness training to cope with grief in chronic pain sufferers (Sagula and Rice, 2004). Authors noted that the source of grief in these patients involved multiple losses related to work, relationships, and other areas of life. All this was complicated by the challenge of living with chronic pain. Subjects were recruited from pain clinic patients seeking psychological help and a total of 71 subjects began the study. A total of 29 women and 10 men were in the treatment group who completed the study with 11 women and 7 men serving as controls. Therapy involved 8 weekly 90-minute sessions and the participants agreed to practice mindfulness meditation once per day. Instruments used included the short form of the Responses to Loss Scale, the Beck Depression Inventory, and the State–Trait Anxiety Inventory.

Results were in predictable directions. The primary hypothesis of this study that the intensity of the two stages of grief (loss issues and growth) would be significantly different between the two groups received partial support. There was a significant difference between the groups on grieving the loss issues. On the issue of growth, the results failed to attain statistical significance between the two groups, although there was evidence of the treatment group benefiting to a greater degree. On the basis of the BDI, the improvement in treatment group was significant compared to the comparison group. This was also true for anxiety, but only on State anxiety. No differences emerged on the Trait anxiety.

This study, one of a kind, provided considerable support for the efficacy of mindfulness meditation in helping cope with grief in a chronic pain population. This study was silent on the question of any effect of this treatment on pain levels. The authors noted that mindfulness enabled the loss issues to be more fully grieved because it promoted a nonjudgmental attitude of emotional and cognitive material, thereby powering defense mechanisms such as intellectualization, rationalization, and denial.

Conclusion

The first point to be noted is that outcome research on grief therapy for chronic illness including chronic pain remains pitiful. On the other hand, if the proposition that grief is grief despite the nature and type of loss, then a preliminary case can be made, drawing on the outcome literature on death and grief therapy, that this indeed is an effective intervention.

Nevertheless, such an extrapolation does not solve the problem of some of the obvious differences between grief experienced as a consequence of chronic illness vis-à-vis death of a loved one. One telling difference is related to the vagaries of chronic disorders. The course is often unpredictable, and is characterized by peaks and valleys. The other critical issue, where grief therapy for the bereaved departs in a significant way from treating grief in chronic pain patients, is the determination of complicated grief in this population. Is our patient John experiencing complicated grief? What are the hallmarks for this condition? This was much less of a problem with Tina, where the grief was related to three deaths, two of them traumatic. She responded well to therapy and antidepressant medication, but over a considerable length of time.

June, on the other hand, presented a more typical picture where her disease flared up, and she reacted with sadness and withdrawal, perhaps even depression. However, grief therapy in her case proved effective. Our last case, John, may be readily recognized by any practitioner in the chronic pain field. The point of note in John's case is his singular inability/unwillingness to accept the consequences of his medical condition or perhaps the medical condition itself. Complicated psychological and personality factors may account for his response to his illness. Grief therapy, predicated on CBT, was marginally effective to the point his level of anger with all and sundry somewhat subsided, and he nominally modified his addiction to physical exertions, which inevitably caused havoc with his pain.

We end this chapter with five observations:

1. The evidence for the efficacy of grief therapy of varying orientations is encouraging;
2. Grief therapy is only effective with complicated grief. In fact, treating normal grief can be harmful;
3. Establishing "complicated grief" in chronic pain sufferers can be problematic;
4. To reiterate, research literature pertaining to the efficacy of grief therapy for chronic medical conditions including chronic pain is not large enough to make any definitive claim;
5. Grief issues among the chronic pain population are common. Redefining identity is a major challenge. Based on two outcome studies for the efficacy of grief therapy for chronic pain sufferers, the picture is encouraging. However, further outcome research is called for before any definitive claims can be made.

References

Allambaugh, D. and Hoyt, W. (1999) Effectiveness of grief therapy: a meta-analysis. J. Couns. Psychol., 46: 370–380.

Alonzo, A. (2000) The experience of chronic illness and post-traumatic stress disorder: the consequences of cumulative adversity. Soc. Sci. Med., 50: 1475–1484.

Bruce, M. (1999) The association between depression and disability. Am. J. Geriatr. Psychiatry, 7: 8–11.

Buttenshaw, P. (1993) Rehabilitation of the elderly lower-limb elderly. Rev. Clin. Gerentol., 3: 69–84.

Chan, E., O'Neil, I., McKenzie, M., Love, A., and Kissane, D. (2004) What works for therapists conducting family meetings: treatment integrity in family focused grief therapy during palliative care and bereavement. J. Pain Symptom Manage., 27: 502–512.

Ellis- Hill, C. and Horn, S. (2000) Change in identity and self-concept: a new theoretical approach to recovery following a stroke. Clin. Rehabil., 14: 279–287.

Esplen, M., Toner, B., Hunter, J., et al. (2000) A supportive-expressive group intervention for women with a family history of breast cancer: results of a phase II study. Psychooncology, 9: 243–252.

Fortner, B (2000) The effectiveness of grief counseling and therapy: a quantitative Review. Dissertation Abstract International. Section B: The Sciences and Engineering, 60(8-B).

Fox, L. and Rau, M. (2001) Augmentative and alternative communication for adults following glossectomy and laryngectomy surgery. Augment. Altern. Commun., 17: 161–166.

Glasscoe, C. and Quittner, A. (2006) Psychological intervention for cystic fibrosis. Cochrane Database Syst. Rev., Issue 3.

Hayashi, T. (1994) Life review process in psychotherapy with the elderly. Hiroshima Forum Psychol., 16: 53–63.

Judd, D. (2001) "To walk the last bit on my own"-narcissistic independence or identification with good objects: issues of loss for a 13 year old boy who had an amputation. J. Child Psychother., 27: 47–67.

Malkinson, R. (2001) Cognitive behavioral therapy and grief and grief: a review and application. Res. Soc. Work Pract., 11: 671–698.

McCullum, M., Piper, W., and Morin, H. (1993) Affect and outcome in short-term therapy for loss. Int. J. Group Psychother., 43: 303–319.

McCallum, M., Piper, W., Ogrodniczuk, J., and Joyce, A. (2003) Relationships among psychological mindedness, alexithymia and outcome in four forms of short-term psychotherapy. Psychol. Psychother., 76: 133–144.

McNeil, D. (2006) Patient, therapist, and observer perspectives on cohesion and alliance and their relationship to outcome in psychodynamic group psychotherapy for persons experiencing complicated grief. Dissertation Abstracts International. Section B: The Sciences and Engineering, 66(10-B).

Nau, D. (1997) Andy writes to his amputated leg: utilizing letter writing as an interventive technique of family grief therapy. J. Fam. Psychother., 8: 1–12.

Neimeyer, R. (1999) Narrative strategies in grief therapy. J. Constructivist Psychol., 12: 65–85.

Neimeyer, R.A. (2000) Searching for the meaning of meaning: grief therapy and the process of reconstruction. Death Stud., 24: 541–558.

Ogrodniczuk, J., Piper, W., and Joyce, A. (2004) Differences in men's and women's responses to short-term group psychotherapy. Psychother. Res., 14: 231–243.

Ogrodniczuk, J., Piper, W., and Joyce, A. (2005) The negative effect of alexithymia on the outcome of group therapy for complicated grief: what role might therapist play? Compr. Psychiatry, 46: 206–213.

Ogrodniczuk, J., Piper, W., Joyce, A., et al. (2002a) Social support as a predictor of response to group therapy for complicated grief. Psychiatry: Interpersonal Biol. Processes, 65: 346–357.

Ogrodniczuk, J., Piper, W., Joyce, A., et al. (2003) NEO-Five factor personality traits as predictors of responses to two forms of group psychotherapy. Int. J. Group Psychother., 53: 417–442.

Ogrodniczuk, J., Piper, W., McCullum, M., et al. (2002b) Interpersonal predictors of group therapy outcome for complicated grief. Int. J. Group Ther., 52: 511–535.

Piper, W., Ogrodniczuk, J., Joyce, A., McCullum, M., and Rosie, J. (2002) Relationship among affect, work and outcome in group therapy for patients with complicated grief. Am. J. Psychother., 56: 347–361.

Piper, W., Ogrodniczuk, J., Lamarche, C., et al. (2005) Level of alliance and outcome in short-term group therapy. Int. J. Group Psychother., 55: 527–550.

Piper, W., Ogrodniczuk, J., McCullum, M., Joyce, A., and Rosie, J. (2003) Expression of affect as a mediator of the relationship between quality of object relations and group therapy outcome for patients with complicated grief. J. Consult. Clin. Psychol., 71: 664–671.

Parkes, M. (1973) Bereavement: Studies if Grief in Adult Life. Harmondsworth: Penguin.

Parkes, M. and Weiss, R. (1983) Recovery from Bereavement. New York, Basic Books.

Rabindranath, K., Daly, C., Butler, L., et al. (2006) Psychosocial interventions for depression in dialysis patients. Cochrane Database Syst. Rev., Issue 3.

Reed, L. (1999) The efficacy of grief therapy as a treatment modality for individuals diagnosed with co-morbid disorders of chronic pain and depression. Dissertation Abstracts International. Section B: Science and Engineering, 59(7-B).

Roy, R. (2001) Social Relations and Chronic Pain. New York, Kluwer Publishing.

Roy, R. (2004) Chronic Pain, Loss and Suffering. Toronto, University of Toronto Press.

Roy, R. (2007) Social dislocation of chronic pain sufferers. In: Bond, M. (Ed.) Encyclopedia of Pain. Berlin/Heidelberg, Springer.

Sagula, D. and Rice, K. (2004) The effectiveness of mindfulness training on the grieving process and emotional well-being of chronic pain patients. J. Clin. Psychol. Med. Settings, 11: 333–342.

Sikkema, K., Hansen, N., Kochman, A., et al. (2004) Outcome from a randomized controlled trial of a group intervention for HIV positive men and women coping with AIDS-related loss and bereavement. Death Stu., 28: 187–209.

Swenson, C. and Fuller, S. (1992) Expression of love, marriage problems, commitment, and anticipatory grief in the marriages of cancer patients. J. Marriage Fam., 54: 191–196.

Thomas, P., Thomas, S., Hillier, C., Galvin, K., and Baker, R. (2006) Psychological interventions for multiple sclerosis. Cochrane Database Syst. Rev. (Issue 3).

Thompson, S. and Kyle, D. (2000) The role of perceived control in coping with the losses associated with chronic illness. In: J. Harvey and E. Miller (Eds.) Loss and Trauma: General and Close Relationship Perspectives (pp. 131–145). New York, Brunner Routledge, Taylor and Francis Group.

Vali, F and Walkup, J (1998) Combined medical and psychological symptoms: impact of disability and healthcare utilization of patients with arthritis. Med. Care, 36: 1073–1084.

Wagner, B., Knaevelsrud, C., and Maercker, A. (2006) Internet-based cognitive-behavioral therapy for complicated grief: a randomized controlled trial. Death Stud., 30: 429–453.

Chapter 7
Brief Therapies

In this chapter a broad category of interventions that fall within the scope of brief therapy are discussed. IPT that we described in Chapter 5 also falls into the brief therapy category, as is CBT—the subject of Chapter 8. In fact, it can be stated with some level of certainty that time-limited brief therapy is the most common method of psychotherapy employed by psychotherapists. Based on the work of several authors, Bor and colleagues (2004) identified the main characteristics of brief therapy, which are as follows:

- The intention is to help move clients to an agreed goal in a time-efficient way; the number of sessions may or may not be specified, although operationally it may be useful to have six to ten sessions in total.
- Time is limited and is used flexibly and creatively.
- The therapist is active throughout the process and a positive, strong, and collaborative alliance is developed.
- Effort is made from the outset to engage the client as early as possible in the therapeutic process. There are clear and achievable goals, and a focus from the outset is maintained.
- The therapist remains flexible and goals may be renegotiated.
- A clear definition of client and therapist responsibilities is achieved.
- Assessment is conducted early and rapidly and is ongoing until the therapy concludes.
- Interventions are introduced promptly.
- Serious problems do not necessarily require profound solutions—small changes may sometimes be sufficient.
- Solutions to problems are co-constructed with clients.
- The client's strengths, abilities, and resources are recognized and encouraged rather than emphasizing pathology.
- Different skills and approaches may be used; the therapist draws on a wide repertoire of skills.
- Change is expected to occur; this expectation may be self-fulfilling; it is also recognized that some change may have already occurred even before therapy gets underway.

R. Roy, *Psychosocial Interventions for Chronic Pain*,
DOI: 10.1007/978-0-387-76296-8_7 © Springer Science+Business Media, LLC 2008

- Change mostly occurs outside the session; termination and expected outcomes are addressed early in therapy and then throughout the therapeutic process; there is a clear sense of ending right from the beginning of therapy.

Arguably, not all of these conditions may be observable in individual cases.

An exception to the abovementioned characteristics is the psychoanalytically or psychodynamically oriented short-term psychotherapies that are predicated on a rather different set of assumptions. Writing on the state of brief therapy, Steenbarger (1994) observed that the question of duration and outcome of therapy was complex. He cited a number of studies that reported weak or nonexistent relationships between these two factors. Furthermore, his review showed that brief therapy was a heterogeneous group of interventions targeted to a broad range of problems and clients. Data showed that psychologically oriented clients were most likely to benefit from brief therapy that was symptom-centered and the goals can be achieved in eight to ten sessions. However, the results were less encouraging for clients with broad, diffuse, and poorly understood patterns where a trusting relationship with the therapist could not be easily achieved. This review concluded that there was no one function linking duration and outcome across all clients, concerns, and helping approaches.

We begin by illustrating the application of task-centered approach (TCA) to treating a chronic pain sufferer. TCA shares similar if not the same characteristics of any brief therapy. This model was developed by two social work academics Reid and Epstein (1972), with its emphasis on "social." In that sense, this model is somewhat a departure from other interventions discussed so far. Action is the foundation of this method and psychosocial problems are rooted in the immediate psychosocial environment of the patient. TCA relies on the "autonomous problem-solving" capacity of the patient. Search is focused on the patient's strength rather than on the psychopathology. Reid and Epstein (1972) proposed a functionally useful classification of problems: (1) interpersonal conflicts; (2) dissatisfaction in social relations; (3) problems with formal organizations; (4) difficulty in role performance; (5) decision-making problems; (6) reactive emotional distress; (7) inadequate resources; and (8) psychosocial or behavioral problems not elsewhere classified. In an update on this model Reid and Fortune (2006) claimed this model to be empirically validated for its efficacy. They presented a number of studies including a few controlled experiments to justify their claim (Dierking et al., 1980; Naleppa and Reid, 1998; Reid and Bailey-Dempsey, 1994; Rzepnicki, 1985). However, none of the studies met the criteria of RCT, and yet the collective weight of the empirical evidence suggested that the claim of efficacy was not without foundation. We now present the case of Thomas.

Thomas, in his late twenties, was referred by his orthopedic surgeon for debilitating neck or shoulder pain. He was a victim of an automobile accident that caused whiplash injury some 8 months prior to his arrival at the pain clinic. His pain had worsened to the point that he could barely cope with day-to-day life. Thomas was a professional engineer and held an excellent position with a small firm. He was having difficulty in functioning in his job, despite a great deal of support from his employer. First, he was placed on sick leave and then let go. He withdrew from all his social activities and found himself in conflict with his only sister, the only relative he had in the city, his very understanding employer, his family physician, an insurance company, and even his close friends.

His job loss was at the top of his concerns. Although single, financial difficulties were beginning to loom large. He had great fear of his benefits running out. His problems as per TCA seemed to be largely in the category of reactive emotional distress. His pain, however, continued unabated. It is also noteworthy that Thomas experienced significant role changes—from a fully functioning adult to chronically ill. The following problems were explicitly agreed upon by Thomas and the therapist:

1. Thomas' withdrawal from social situation;
2. His falling out with his only sister;
3. Unemployment and financial concerns; and
4. Dissatisfaction with his lawyer for his inaction.

It must be noted that none of the problems involved any pain-related issues.

Agreement was reached between the patient and the therapist on the following goals:

1. Plan to socialize;
2. Make-up with his sister;
3. Meetings with the lawyer and the landlord to work on Thomas' concerns; and
4. Realistic plans to return to work.

A contract for ten therapy sessions of an hour's duration over 3 months was agreed upon. The action plan was:

1. Thomas would make a point of going out with his best friend at least once a week. He would also do his grocery shopping once a week;
2. He would call his sister and resolve his conflict and meet with her at least once a week;
3. A meeting with his lawyer was arranged and he was to report back to the therapist on the outcome. A similar meeting was arranged with the landlord; and
4. Thomas would postpone any thoughts of returning to work in the immediate future.

Pain was made a non-negotiable problem as it was unlikely that pain would be completely alleviated. This last point was critical because Thomas had to take charge of his life despite the pain, and not wait for its alleviation. The pain issues were between him and the physicians, and not part of the psychotherapy process.

The path of therapy with Thomas could be best described as jagged. Part of the reason was Thomas' propensity to invoke his pain and the fact that so little progress was being made on that front. His motivation flagged from time to time. He was terrified of confronting his lawyer. By and large, however, he adhered to the plan.

His reconciliation with his sister was achieved in short order. This was his first major achievement. It restored some of his confidence. Resumption of his friendships also had similar effect. Thomas' assumptive world was being slowly restored.

A singular fact of life for many chronic pain patients is their sense of loss of autonomy and control over their lives. Hence, it is critical to rank-order the tasks. For Thomas getting reconnected with his sister was the simplest, but in terms of restoring some of Thomas' lost confidence, this achievement was significant. Thomas succeeded in realizing all his goals albeit on a slower pace, than originally agreed upon. The last task was related to employment. After about a year after the formal termination of therapy, he obtained employment with an automobile manufacturer at a very high salary.

TCA is a short-term, goal-oriented therapy, and behavior-based approach. Its merit lies in the fact that from the very outset, the patient is responsible for the outcome of therapy. The task-development process in itself is of considerable therapeutic value. The message to the patient is unambiguous: "You are capable of taking charge of your life." In the following pages we review the efficacy of brief therapy (1) in general and (2) in relation to medically ill and chronic pain patients.

Brief Therapy and Outcome

We begin by examining two major reviews on the outcome of brief psychotherapy. First, a meta-analytic review of short-term dynamically oriented psychotherapy (STDT) (Anderson and Lambert, 1995), and second, a review of outcome research for solution-focused brief therapy (Gingerich and Eisengart, 2000).

Anderson and Lambert (1995) included studies that met the following criteria: (1) at least one treatment group was designated by the authors of the study as either psychodynamic or psychoanalytic; (2) comparison with a no-treatment control group, or an alternative therapy; (3) treatment which lasted 40 sessions (which does not strictly fit into the brief category) or less; (4) samples comprising of non-psychotic outpatients; and (5) provision of data to compute effect sizes (ES). A total of 26 studies met the criteria. Studies were divided for the purpose of analysis into three groups: (1) STDT vs no treatment; (2) STDT vs minimal treatment; and (3) STDT vs alternative treatment.

Results showed that the average effect size (ES) over the 11 studies that compared STDT to no treatment was 0.57. However, ESs were quite heterogeneous and not well represented by the composite ES. This problem resulted from relatively poor outcome with STDT for psychosomatic conditions. They were more difficult to treat.

In the second category of STDT versus minimal treatment, no firm conclusions could be reached due to only five studies in this category. STDT produced significant ES in some situations (assessing general or target symptoms), but not in others (assessing somatic symptoms or social adjustment).

In the final category of STDT versus alternative treatment, which included 18 studies, there was no evidence of STDT being better or worse than other forms of interventions. However, STDT outperformed alternative therapies in the following cases: when assessment focused on personality functioning, when patients were addicted to drugs, when manuals were used and when therapists were trained in STDT. The authors concluded that STDT produced ES comparable to those achieved by other forms of therapy. One point of note is that 40 sessions or less, which was the length of intervention for STDT in this review, may not be regarded as particularly short term. Steenbarger (1994) noted that conventionally brief therapies range between 12 and 25 sessions, and not infrequently even less than that.

Our next review is of a report on 15 outcome studies related to solution-focused brief therapy (Gingerich and Eisengart, 2000). Solution-focused brief therapy (SFBT) is a popular therapeutic approach that focuses on constructions of solutions rather than the more traditional problem-solving approach. This review examined the outcome of 15 controlled studies to determine the extent of empirical support for SFBT. Articles reviewed included all controlled studies in English literature up to and including 1999. The term "controlled studies" was used to include studies that employed a comparison group or single-case repeated-measure design. Based on the quality, these studies were divided into three categories: (1) five well-controlled studies; (2) four moderately controlled; and (3) six poorly controlled.

The five well-controlled studies included (1) depression in college students; (2) parenting skills; (3) rehabilitation of orthopedic patients (we shall review this study in detail in the following section); (4) recidivism in prison population; and (5) antisocial adolescent offenders. This brief list suggests application of SFT with a wide-ranging set of problems. To this can be added the studies in the moderately controlled studies, which included (1) counseling high school students; (2) solution-focused school groups; (3) SFBT training for mental health supervisors; and (4) couples therapy. In the category of poorly controlled studies the problems reported were just as varied.

The authors came to the following conclusions:

- That given the methodological problems in many of the 15 studies, arriving at definitive conclusions was not possible.
- The five well-controlled studies, however, showed clear benefit of SFBT. However, these studies did not compare SFBT with another treatment, which raised questions about the specific influence of SFBT versus general attention effects.
- All the studies were conducted by advocates of SFBT, and in some instances SFBT was implemented by the authors themselves, raising the question of bias.

The current studies fell short of clearly establishing the efficacy of SFBT, but provided preliminary support for this method of intervention. We now review a few selected recent (since 2000) outcome studies that include a few reports on the outcome of SFBT.

One recent study compared SFBT with cognitive therapy for their efficacy in treating adult patients attending a clinical psychology service (Rothwell, 2005). This was a retrospective study using pseudo-randomization. Data was extracted retrospectively from the database of a clinical psychology service operation. This database contained client information routinely collected by therapists. All referrals were made by the local family physicians. Any client intervention that identified SFBT or CBT as the sole therapeutic intervention was included in this study. The sample thus identified consisted of 119 in the CBT group and 41 in SFBT group. Clients from the top of the waiting list were allocated to the first therapist who had an appointment slot available, regardless of the type of problems or other factors. The choice of therapy was made by the therapist.

Results showed that SFBT was indeed shorter that CBT and the difference was accounted for by single-session attenders, which is consistent with the brief therapy approach. SFBT clients were seen for two sessions on average compared to five for CBT. A simple therapist-rated outcome scale failed to find any significant difference. It is noteworthy that this was a small study with several limitations. First, the SFBT clients were seen, almost exclusively, by one therapist who was also the author. CBT clients were seen by several therapists, thus raising the possibility of a confounding factor. As noted earlier, the groups were not systematically randomized. In short, this study failed to overcome some of the methodological shortcoming noted in the preceding section.

Our second study was more in the nature of a follow-up assessment of outcome a year after patients terminated SFBT in an outpatient mental health clinic (Macdonald, 2005). The author described this study as an uncontrolled naturalistic outcome study in a National Health Service (UK) Mental Health Trust. Thus, it has many limitations. A questionnaire was sent to clients and their family doctors 1 year after they ceased to attend. "Good outcome" was defined as either clients themselves reporting that they had achieved their goals or the family physicians that goals were achieved, if no information was directly available from the clients. The sample reported here comprised of 75 clients, of whom 53 were seen and 41 traced at follow-up. Thirty-one (76%) reported a good outcome, with an average of just over five sessions; 20% attending only one session. This data was combined from previous studies which produced 170 referrals of whom 136 attended and 118 were traced. Good outcome was reported by 83 clients (70%), with a mean of four sessions per case. This study falls in the category of a clinical follow-up study completely lacking in any rigor in terms of outcome measures. In methodological terms, this was a very poorly designed investigation, and no firm conclusion can be drawn as far as efficacy of SFBT is concerned.

Our final report on the efficacy of SFBT examined the role of working alliance in influencing outcome in brief interpersonal (BIT) therapy and SFBT (Wettersten et al., 2005). Authors noted that while working alliance is a critical component of BIT, that is not so in relation to SFBT. A total of 26 therapist–clients dyads completed SFBT at a university-based clinic. The agency had a 12-session limit, with therapy ranging from 3 to 12 sessions. As for BIT, archival data from a previously published study was used for comparison. Altogether 38 patients completed BIT. Development of strong working alliance was emphasized. Though the model followed was described as a brief therapy approach, some patients were seen for up to 48 sessions. Clients from both groups were carefully matched in collecting data from patients who received BIT.

One of the striking findings of this study was there was no significant relationship between working alliance and outcome in relation to SFBT. On the other hand, this association was significant with BIT. There were no differences in patients' level of psychological distress, their satisfaction with counseling, and their rating of working alliance between SFBT and BIT. Although the purpose of this study was not designed to test efficacy of BIT and SFBT, the main conclusion did find the two models to be equally effective in treating psychologically distressed individuals. This was not an RCT and the comparison group was, in fact, drawn from archival sources. Furthermore, BIT did not strictly adhere to "brief" intervention, thus raising questions about the validity of comparing two brief interventions.

One inescapable conclusion is that more recent outcome studies of SFBT have failed to improve on the earlier studies. This is despite growing popularity with its emphasis on efficiency and brevity. Wettersten and associates (2005) noted that there were, in fact, rather few studies that tested the effectiveness of SFBT. Many had serious methodological shortcomings, although some did demonstrate evidence of effectiveness of SFBT. SFBT awaits methodologically sound studies to determine its efficacy.

We turn our attention now to examining two more outcome studies of brief therapy using varied techniques. The first involved assessing the efficacy of brief psychodynamic interpersonal therapy (PIT) to treat self-poisoning patients (Guthrie et al., 2003). To that end, patients presenting at an emergency department in Manchester, UK, with deliberate self-poisoning were randomly assigned to PIT or usual care. Patients were assigned to the two treatment conditions in blocks (of 12 consecutive patients) using randomization lists provided by a statistician. Assessments were carried out at baseline, following the treatment phase of 4 weeks and at 6-month follow-up. Patients were offered four sessions of PIT. Therapy was administered by three nurse-therapists in patient's home. Fifty-eight patients received PIT, and 61, the usual treatment. The main outcome measure was the Beck Scale for Suicidal Ideation and the Beck Depression Inventory. Four sessions of PIT for deliberate self-poisoning was found to be effective in reducing suicidal ideation in patients with less severe depression, no prior history of self-harm, and who did not consume alcohol with the overdose. It is noteworthy that the regression models used accounted for 40% of the variance, which meant that many other factors not investigated influenced outcome. This was a well-designed and executed study, and the conclusion was that patients with less severe psychiatric history were likely to benefit from PIT.

The final review to be discussed in this section examined application of brief therapy for clients with mild-to-moderate alcohol dependence (Adamson et al., 2004). This study was an RCT to test the efficacy of motivational enhancement therapy (MET). One hundred and twenty two patients with alcohol dependence were randomly assigned to three different forms of brief therapy, based on their choice, which were four sessions of MET, four sessions of non-directive reflective listening (NDRL), and a no further counseling option. Treatment outcome was measured with two key factors, one focused on drinking and the other on global functioning.

Results showed that there was no difference in either outcome or treatment process according to whether or not patients were allocated to their choice of therapy. Authors noted that this key finding served to reassure that RCTs were ethical in that they did not, by the very nature of absence of choice, impaired treatment outcome. Overall, the sample showed a significant reduction in unequivocal drinking from baseline to follow-up. Furthermore, MET was found to be significantly more effective in reducing unequivocal heavy drinking than either NDRL or no further counseling. There were no significant differences between the latter two. This was a very well designed, somewhat novel study which gave patients the choice of therapy, demonstrating the superiority of a short-term therapeutic intervention (MET), and also addressing some questions related to the randomization process.

These two studies are methodologically acceptable with randomized controlled groups which clearly demonstrated superiority of brief therapy with two rather divergent clinical populations. However, within the category of brief therapy two rather conceptually different treatment approaches were reported. This remains a key issue in terms of evaluating efficacy of brief therapy. Brief therapy appears in many guises and employed with an extraordinary array of problems which makes it somewhat challenging to draw definitive conclusions.

Brief Therapy and Chronic Pain and Medically Ill Patients

Reports of psychological interventions for medically ill patients abound. Behavioral and more specifically CBT are the most commonly reported therapies. We have excluded that body of literature from this section as we devote the next chapter to CBT. It must be stated at the outset that outcome studies of brief therapy used to treat patients with organic diseases or even psychosomatic disorders are very sparse. A very recent book on evidence-based psychotherapy confirms this observation (Fisher and O'Donohue, 2006). However, this book contains one chapter on chronic pain and another on irritable bowel syndrome. We shall presently discuss these two reports. Even clinical reports are few and far between. Application of brief therapy in the medical context may not be a common occurrence. Our literature search showed that much of that literature is devoted to making a case for brief therapy rather than demonstrating its effectiveness. Nevertheless, we were able to find a few reports which we shall report below.

One clinical report discussed an 8-year-old girl and her 13-year-old brother who were successfully treated for encropesis without ever being seen in therapy (Shapiro and Henderson, 1992). SFBT was used with their father, and only after four sessions the encropesis was resolved. Apparently, a change in the father's behavior, which meant being more involved in the lives of his children, rather than a change in the children's led to this dramatic outcome.

This report relied solely on the feedback by the father as to the outcome. Although the authors went to some length to explain the reasons for the successful outcome and how only four sessions yielded the results that therapy did, yet, in the absence of objective measures, the success of this case has to be viewed with caution. The authors themselves acknowledge that reasons for reporting this case was its success, but they also recognized the need for ascertaining the efficacy of brief therapy models. In a personal communication to the authors, the proponent of SFBT, deShazer maintained that "unsuccessful cases are not related to the type of presenting complaint or any other factors except that failure may be related to the therapist and the client having different goals for therapy". This is a factual observation and a prerequisite for successful outcome. Yet, it is just one predictor of outcome among many. This clinical report must be seen for what it is. It is anecdotal and as such provides an interesting hypothesis that remains to be tested.

Another report of brief therapy outcome involving 21 children, aged between 1 and 6 at first consultation and 4–10 at the time of the study with somatic or behavioral problems, reported remission of symptoms in 92% of the patients (Maestro et al., 1997). Patients were divided into three groups: without disorders; mild psychopathological disorder; and serious psychopathological disorder. A strong correlation was found between precocious mother–child relationship and the therapy outcome for the children.

The third report described the application of solution-focused brief therapy (SFBT) in a family medicine setting in Seoul, Korea (Park, 1997). They observed that SFBT was a suitable therapy to support families with a whole range of psychosocial and medical problems in a university department of family medicine. The majority of the problems were in the psychosomatic category, distress around a chronically family member, or the death of a family member. Other problems noted were severe illness, family violence or abuse. Two cases were described: one involving a 38-year-old man with frequent bowel movement and lower abdominal pain and the second case involved a 32-year-old woman with "swirling dizziness attacks." Both these cases responded well to SFBT.

The effectiveness of brief therapy was demonstrated in treating victims of an earthquake who had developed chronic post-traumatic stress disorder by short-term behavior therapy (Basaglu et al., 2003). Given the magnitude of mental health problems following a major natural disaster, authors devised a brief cost-effective intervention. Altogether, 231 consecutive referrals were assigned to five locations for therapy 13 months after a major earthquake. Treatment consisted of self-exposure instructions based on enhancement of sense of control. The survivors received a mean of 4.3 sessions. Multiple measures were used and significant treatment effects and clinically meaningful effect sizes were noted on all measures. A dramatic 76% of the patients reported improvement after only one session and this was raised to 88% after the second session. At follow-up of a sub-sample at 1–2 months and 3–9 months, initial improvement was maintained. This study is of particular value as it demonstrated the efficacy of what can only be termed as minimal intervention.

Rosser and associates (1983) reported a study of the outcome of brief psychotherapy with patients disabled by chronic obstructive pulmonary disease (COPD). Forty-three men and 22 women with severe COPD were randomly allocated for 8 weeks to one of three types of psychotherapy or to an unrelated control group, and were followed up 6 months later. Psychotherapy consisted of eight 45-minute sessions, which were tape-recorded and transcribed. Treatment groups consisted of:

(1) the analytic group from two psychoanalysts using transference interpretations;
(2) the supportive group from the same two therapists but withholding transference;
(3) the nurse group focusing on practical management of the disease;
(4) control group without psychotherapy, but biweekly laboratory tests.

Results were complex. Those receiving treatment from the nurses improved most on dyspnea, but showed less improvement on the psychological measures. The group receiving supportive therapy showed most improvement on the psychological measures. The authors noted that the nurse and the supportive techniques demanded an active concentration on the patient as a person. In contrast, the analytic technique created some distance between the therapists and the patients by the virtue of a dispassionate posture of the therapists. Psychoanalytic approach proved to be least effective in this trial.

Our final report is a randomized trial of lifestyle modification to treat obesity, which included teaching patients to control the external environment involving diet, exercise, and behavior therapy, and pharmacotherapy, using siburtramine (Wadden et al., 2005). Lifestyle modification counseling was the method chosen along with pharmacotherapy to treat obesity in 224 obese adults, who were randomly assigned to receive 15 mg of siburtramine per day, delivered by a primary healthcare provider in 8 visits of to 10–15 minutes each; lifestyle modification counseling alone, delivered in 30 group sessions (hardly in the brief therapy category); drug plus 30 group sessions of life-style counseling (combined therapy); and groups who received a combination of the drug and counseling delivered by a primary healthcare provider in 8 visits of 10–15 minutes each. A total of 55 subjects were assigned to the lifestyle counseling alone, who attended weekly meetings from week 1 to 18. From weeks 20 to 40, these groups met biweekly, and a follow-up at week 52. Groups consisted of 7–10 subjects and the sessions lasted 90 minutes. Results were in the predictable direction in that subjects who received combined therapy lost most weight and those who received the drug alone, the least weight. Weight loss was noted in all groups.

One inescapable conclusion has to be that the efficacy of brief therapy in the context of medical disorders remains an open question, and the data that exists fail to provide any evidence to its usefulness. However, our last study does conclusively show that brief therapy in conjunction with medical treatment can be very effective.

Reports on the efficacy of brief therapy for treatment of chronic pain conditions are few and far between. A few clinical reports exist on the use of brief therapy that include "therapeutic release of suppressed emotion," anger in this case in combination with acupuncture. This technique was used with a male adult suffering from chronic pain (Williamson, 2002). Clinical outcome in routine evaluation forms were used both before and after 2 weeks after the termination of therapy and showed a dramatic change to normalization, which was maintained at a 4 week follow-up.

Another report makes a case for the Eriksonian principles in the use of brief therapy with chronic pain sufferers (Feldman, 1997). This approach combines a body–mind healing perspective and can be integrated into a multi-disciplinary team approach to pain management.

Different types of brief therapy have been tested with irritable bowel syndrome, a very painful chronic pain disorder. Short-term psychodynamic psychotherapy (Creed et al., 2003; Guthrie et al., 1991, 1995; Svedlund, 1983) , IPT (chapter 5), relaxation response meditation (Keefer and Blanchard, 2002) and progressive muscle relaxation alone (Blanchard et al., 1993) have all been demonstrated to have some positive results in terms of more effective coping with this very painful condition.

Cockburn and associates (1997) evaluated the impact of SFBT on psychosocial adjustment and return to work for patients with orthopedic injuries. Forty-eight patients and their partners were referred for work-re-entry program. Patients were first-time recipients of worker's compensation and their partners were in full-time employment. As for injuries, 73% had spinal injuries or injuries in their upper extremities.

Subjects were randomly assigned to one of four groups. The treatment groups consisted of groups 1 and 3 and the intervention consisted of 6 weekly 1 hour sessions of SFBT plus the standard rehabilitation program. The control groups, 2 and 4, received only the standard rehabilitation program. On the all the measures of psychosocial functioning such as acquiring social support, reframing of the problems, and mobilizing the family, the treatment groups scored significantly higher than the control groups. Most strikingly, more than 68% of subjects in the treatment groups returned to work within 7 days from the completion of treatment. Only 4% of the control groups managed to return to work. This study clearly demonstrated the value of addressing critical social issues that may enhance patient's coping with pain and disability. Research method employed by this study was a rigorous, randomized design that used a treatment manual and standardized outcome measures. SFBT was demonstrated to be a very effective therapy with this population.

Leichsenring (2005) reviewed the empirical evidence for the efficacy of psycho-dynamic and psychoanalytic therapies. He noted that psychoanalytic therapy did not lend itself to RCTs and had severe limitations as an absolute standard. Studies of psychodynamic psychotherapy published between 1960 and 2004 were identi-fied through a computerized search using Medline. Twenty-two RCTs providing evidence of the efficacy of psychodynamic psychotherapy were identified. Four of these studies related to somatoform disorder, which in this case was exclusively irritable bowel syndrome, which we report below. The major conclusions reached by this review were: (1) psychoanalytic therapy was more effective than no therapy or treatment as usual; and (2) psychoanalytic therapy was more effective that shorter forms of psychodynamic therapy.

Several authors have reported on the effectiveness of psychodynamic psychother-apy in the treatment of IBS (Creed et al., 2003; Guthrie et al., 1991; Svedlund, 1983). Svedlund (1983) reported on 101 IBS patients, who had been ill for at least a year and attending an outpatient clinic, who were randomly assigned to two treatment groups. Both groups received the same medical treatment, but the experimental group ($n = 50$) also received dynamically oriented short-term psychotherapy which consisted of ten 1-hour sessions spread over a period of 3 months. Outcome mea-sures comprised of changes in the severity of symptoms, social adjustment, and coping ability with problems. Assessments were made at intake, 3 months after the completion of psychotherapy, and at 1-year follow-up.

Initial results indicated improvement in both groups during treatment, but at the 3-month follow-up psychotherapy group demonstrated significantly greater improvement. At the 1-year follow-up, the psychotherapy group showed further improvement, while the control group showed some deterioration. On measures of severity by independent raters, almost 50% of patients in the psychotherapy group reported improvement at follow-up versus 10% in the control group. On the self-rating scales, 75% of the psychotherapy group reported improvement opposed to 40% in the control group.

Superiority of the combined treatment was apparent the end of the therapy program, but became more pronounced after 1-year follow-up. Significantly greater improvement was noted in cases of abdominal pain, bowel dysfunction, indigestion, and dyspepsia; depressive symptoms, sleep disturbance, and sexual interest; social and leisure life, general distress, coping with work, and marriage relations.

Patients with high expectation of improvement, and patients with dyspepsia and a need for deference and aggression were less suitable for psychotherapy. In addition, a need for achievement and a higher social class predicted positive outcome for psychotherapy. Suitability for insight-oriented psychotherapy was related to coping ability than to symptomatic improvement. The effectiveness of brief psychodynamic psychotherapy was shown to be highly effective in the treatment of a rather painful and intractable chronic disease.

Guthrie and associates (1991) in a study of 100 patients with irritable bowel syndrome reported the benefits of short-term psychodynamic psychotherapy, relaxation, and standard medical treatment, but they had failed to respond to standard treatment during the preceding 6 months. In a controlled trial, these patients were compared to patients who received standard medical intervention. At 3 months, the treatment group showed significantly greater improvement than the controls on the physicians' as well as the patients' ratings of diarrhea and abdominal pain. There was, however, no improvement on constipation. Factors that predicted positive outcome included overt psychiatric symptoms and intermittent pain exacerbate by stress. Those with constant pain were only marginally helped. Psychotherapy proved to be feasible and effective in two-thirds of patients suffering from irritable bowel syndrome who had failed to respond to standard medical treatment.

Creed and associates (2003) also demonstrated the effectiveness of short-term psychodynamic psychotherapy in the treatment of irritable bowel syndrome. Compared to routine care, psychotherapy was found to be significantly more effective and was at least as effective as medication (Paroxetine). The sample consisted of 257 subjects recruited from 7 hospitals. Fifty-nine of 85 patients (69%) were randomized to psychotherapy and 43 out of 86 patients (50%) of the paroxetine group completed the treatment.

Both treatments were found to be superior to "as usual" therapy in improving the physical aspects of health related quality of life, but there were no significant differences on the psychological measures. However during the follow-up year, psychotherapy but not paroxetine was associated with a significant reduction in healthcare costs compared with treatment as usual. The authors concluded that for patients with severe irritable bowel syndrome, both paroxetine and psychotherapy improved health-related quality of life at no additional cost.

Keefer and Blanchard (2004) in their chapter on psychological treatment for IBS noted that cognitive behavioral interventions have been the most commonly used interventions in the treatment of IBS. They noted that few other forms of treatment, such as interpersonal psychotherapy, dynamic psychotherapy (discussed above), relaxation response meditation (Keefer and Blanchard, 2002), and hypnotherapy (Gonsalkorale et al., 2002), were also shown to have some degree of effectiveness in treating this complex disorder. Gatchel and associates (2004) in their chapter on evidence-based therapy for chronic pain reported exclusively on CBT as the treatment of choice.

Conclusion

It will not be an exaggeration to state that brief therapy, regardless of the type and orientation, is the most common mode of psychotherapy practiced today. It is, by and large, effective and economical. Besides, all the evidence points in the direction that brief therapy is more effective than long-term psychodynamic psychotherapy, which is usually rooted in Freudian or neo-Freudian perspectives.

Although there is some consensus about the definition of brief therapy in terms of its length, much flexibility can be detected within the framework. We reported on one study that could involve as many as 40 sessions , while in reality patients used much less. However, in practice most brief therapy entails 6–12 sessions.

In this chapter, we took somewhat of an arbitrary approach to report on the types of brief therapy which may not be in regular use in medical and pain clinic settings. To that end, we examined the effectiveness of SFBT, which has gained widespread popularity among practitioners, only to discover that evidence of its success in treating medical conditions is somewhat wanting. Our review of the outcome studies with SFBT attests to that fact. Nevertheless, until well-designed controlled studies are carried out, we must suspend our judgment.

The next significant approach we reported involved brief psychodynamic psychotherapy, and here we did find a number of well-designed studies, albeit, somewhat small in number. These studies investigated the effectiveness of this particular therapy with irritable bowel syndrome, which is somewhat of a limitation. It must also be acknowledged that application of psychodynamic psychotherapy in the treatment of medically ill patients may not be in wide use. In fact, it can be said with some confidence based on literature search that it is rarely the treatment of choice in pain clinic settings. Nevertheless, brief psychodynamic psychotherapy appears to provide an effective alternative to the more commonly used behavioral approaches in pain clinic settings.

References

Adamson, S., Sellman, J., and Gore, G. (2004) Therapy preference and treatment outcome in clients with mild to moderate alcohol dependence. Drug Alcohol Rev., 209–216.

Anderson, E. and Lambert, M. (1995) Short-term dynamically oriented psychotherapy: a review and meta-analysis. Clin. Psychol. Rev., 15: 503–514.

Basaglu, M., Livanou, M., Salciogly, E., and Kalender, D. (2003) A brief behavioral treatment of chronic post-traumatic stress disorder in earthquake survivors: results from an open clinical trial. Psychol. Med., 33: 647–654.

Blanchard, E., Greene, B., Schrff, L., and Schwarz-McMorris, S. (1993) Relaxation training as a treatment for irritable bowel syndrome. Biofeedback Self Regul., 18: 125–132.

Bor, R., Gill, S., Miller, R., and Parrott, C. (2004) Doing Therapy Briefly. Houndmills, Hampshire, UK, Palgrave Macmillan.

Cockburn, J., Thomas, F., and Cockburn, O. (1997) Solution-focused therapy and psychosocial adjustments to orthopedic rehabilitation in a work-hardening program. J. Occup. Rehabil., 7: 97–106.

Creed, F., Fernandes, L., Guthrie, E., et al. (2003) The cost-effectiveness of psychotherapy and paroxetine for severe irritable bowel syndrome. Gastroenterology, 124: 303–317.

Dierking, B., Brown, M., and Fortune, A. (1980) Task-centered treatment in a residential facility for the elderly: a clinical trial. J. Gerontol. Soc. Work, 2: 225–240.

Feldman, J. (1997) Rehabilitation of chronic pain patients: expanding an Eriksonian approach to interdisciplinary team treatment. In: Matthews, W. and Edgette, J. (Eds.) Current Thinking and Research in Brief Therapy: Solutions, Strategies, Narratives, Vol. 1, pp. 1354–1367. Philadelphia, PA, Brunner/Mazel.

Gatchel, R., Robinson, R., and Stowell, A. (2004) Psychotherapy with chronic pain patients. In: Fisher, J. and O' Donohue, W. (Eds.) (2006) Practitioner's Guide to Evidence Based Practice. New York, Springer

Gonsalkorale, W., Houghton, L.A., and Whorwell, P. (2002) Hypnosis in irritable bowel syndrome: a large scale audit of a clinical service with examination of factors influencing responsiveness. Am. J. Gastroenterol., 97: 954–961.

Gingerich, W. and Eisengart, S. (2000) Solution-focused brief therapy: a review of the outcome research. Fam. Process, 39: 477–490.

Guthrie, E., Creed, F., Dawson, D., and Tomenson, B. (1991) A controlled trial of psychological treatment of irritable bowel syndrome. Gastroenterology, 100: 450–457.

Guthrie, E., Kapur, N., Mackway-Jones, K., et al. (1995) Randomised controlled trial of brief psychological intervention after deliberate self poisoning. BMJ, 323: 135–139.

Guthrie, E., Kapur, N., Mackway-Jones, K., et al. (2003) Predictors of outcome following psychodynamic-interpersonal therapy for deliberate self-poisoning. Aust. N Z J. Psychiatry, 37: 532–536.

Keefer, L. and Blanchard, E. (2002) A one-year follow-up of relaxation response meditation on the symptoms of irritable bowel syndrome: results of a controlled trial study. Behav. Res. Ther., 40: 541–546.

Keefer, L. and Blanchard, E. (2004) Irritable bowel syndrome. In: Fisher, J. and O' Donohue, W. (Eds.) Practitioner's Guide to Evidence-Based Psychotherapy. New York, Springer.

Leichsenring, F. (2005) Are psychodynamic and psychoanalytic therapies effective? A review of empirical data. Int. J. Psychoanal., 86: 841–868.

Macdonald, A. (2005) Brief therapy in adult psychiatry: results from fifteen years of practice. J. Fam. Ther., 27: 65–75.

Maestro, S., Muratori, F., Tosi, B., and Viglione, V. (1997) The outcome for precocious psychosomatic and behavioral disorders. Giornale di Neuropsichiatria dell'Eta Evolutiva, 17: 22–33.

Naleppa, M. and Reid, W. (1998) Task-centered case management for the elderly: developing a practice model. Res. Soc. Work Pract., 8: 63–85.

Park, EunSook. (1997) An application of brief therapy to family medicine. Contemp. Fam. Ther., 19: 81–88.

Reid, W. and Bailey-Dempsey, C. (1994) Content analysis in design and development. Res. Soc. Work Pract., 4: 101–114.

Reid, W. and Epstein, L. (Eds.) (1972) Task-Centered Casework. New York, Columbia University Press.

Reid, W. and Fortune, A. (2006) Task-centered practice: an exemplar of evidence-based practice. In: Roberts, A. and Yeager, K. (Eds.) Foundations of Evidence-Based Social Work Practice. New York, Oxford University Press.

Rosser, R., Denford, J., Heslop. A., et al. (1983) Breathlessness and psychiatric morbidity in chronic bronchitis and emphysema: a study of psychotherapeutic management. Psychol. Med., 13: 93–110.

Rothwell, N. (2005) How brief is solution focused brief therapy. Clin. Psychol. Psychother., 12: 402–405.

Rzepnicki, T. (1985) Task-centered interventions in foster care services. In: Fortune, A. (Ed.) Task-Centered Practice with Families and Groups (pp. 172–184). New York, Springer.

Shapiro, L. and Henderson, J. (1992) Brief therapy for encropesis: a case study. J. Fam. Psychother., 3: 1–12.

Steenbarger, B. (1994) Duration and outcome in psychotherapy: an integrative view. Prof. Psychol. Res. Pr., 25: 111–119.

Svedlund, J.G. (1983) Psychotherapy in irritable model syndrome: a controlled outcome study. Acta Psychiatr. Scand., 67: 7–86.

Wadden, T., Berkowitz, R., Womble, L., et al. (2005) Randomized trial of lifestyle modification and pharmacotherapy for obesity. N. Engl. J. Med., 353: 2111–2120.

Wettersten, K., Lichtenberg, J., and Mallinckrodt, B. (2005) Associations between working alliance and outcome in solution-focused therapy and brief interpersonal therapy. Psychother. Res., 15: 33–43.

Williamson, A. (2002) Chronic psychosomatic pain alleviated by brief therapy. Contemp. Hypnosis, 19: 118–124.

Chapter 8
Cognitive Behavioral Therapy

Cognitive behavioral therapy (CBT) has been rigorously subjected to RCTs and has been shown to be very effective in the treatment of a wide variety of psychological disorders. It is probably the most frequently used method of psychotherapy in the treatment of chronic pain sufferers. The landmark book by Turk et al. (1983) laid the foundation for the application of CBT in the treatment of chronic pain sufferers. Since then there have been abundant reports of successful outcome for this therapy. We shall presently review some of the more recent outcome literature. It will not be an exaggeration to state that CBT has achieved the status of one of the most, if not the most, effective psychological therapies in treating chronic pain sufferers. Yet, our review will show that CBT yields a mixed outcome and awaits further validation.

Five assumptions underlie the use of this therapy in chronic pain patients (Turk, 2002):

(1) People are active processors of information unlike passive reactors to environmental contingencies.
(2) A person's thoughts do impact on emotion-eliciting and physiological arousal-eliciting behavior.
(3) The behavior is reciprocally determined by both the environment and the individual.
(4) Interventions designed to alter behavior should emphasize maladaptive thoughts and behaviors.
(5) People are active agents of change of their maladaptive modes of responding.

Beyond these assumptions, four goals of CBT have been identified for the management of chronic pain (Holzman et al., 1986):

(1) Enable patients to believe that they can manage their pain.
(2) Help chronic pain sufferers to learn to identify and monitor their thoughts, feelings, and behaviors and understand how these phenomena are interrelated.
(3) Help develop appropriate behaviors to cope more effectively with pain.
(4) Maintain the improvements gained during therapy beyond the active treatment phase and incorporate them in their daily management of pain.

R. Roy, *Psychosocial Interventions for Chronic Pain*,
DOI: 10.1007/978-0-387-76296-8_8 © Springer Science+Business Media, LLC 2008

CBT has four major components to achieve the above goals:

(1) reconceptualization;
(2) skills acquisition;
(3) skills consolidation; and
(4) generalization and maintenance (Turk and Gatchell, 2002).

At this point we present two cases to demonstrate (1) a successful outcome of CBT in the case of a headache sufferer and (2) a more mixed picture in the case of a patient with a complex medical history and pain.

Anita, a middle-aged school teacher, presented at a pain clinic with a history of severe headaches. Over the years she had received varied diagnoses for her head pain and finally it was diagnosed as tension headache. Her history of headache dated back to her early thirties. She had learned to cope quite well, and the pain generally responded well to standard treatment for head pain. However, over the past year or so, her pain had worsened and she was taking more and more time off work. She would be away from work for as many as 7 or 8 days per month. Her past medical history was complex and included back surgery to decompress C6 nerve roots. The surgery was successful, but her headaches worsened following her surgery.

Anita was single and work was at the very center of her life. She loved teaching and was highly valued by her peers and students. She had many friends and engaged in various activities. Of late, those activities had come to a virtual halt. She was afraid of going out in case her headache got worse. At the point of her inception at the pain clinic, she had continuous headache that became quite unbearable at the end of her school day. She had almost learned to expect her headache getting worse during the evening hours. She described herself as a very tense person and did not quite know how to relax. However, it must be noted that despite her headaches, she was still a high-functioning individual. She was on antidepressant medication, in addition to Tylenol 3 and Codeine Contin, which she used for breakthrough pain.

At the end of her psychosocial assessment, Anita was offered six sessions of CBT, which she accepted. Therapy focused on reconceptualization and relaxation. The fact that she was highly intelligent and high-functioning was constantly reinforced during therapy. She was asked to practice relaxation at the end of her school day. During the second session she reported that relaxation had helped to curb her anxiety, and at the end of the day she was far less apprehensive of getting bad headaches. In the ensuing weekly therapy sessions, her level of mastery over pain was clearly on the rise. She had not missed a single day of school in the preceding 4 weeks. She also reported that she was far less anxious and she was getting "very good" at relaxing. There was a 40% reduction in her intake of medicine for her breakthrough pain. At the time of writing, she continues to function well and her headache has greatly subsided. She has been scheduled for a review in 8 weeks.

Our next case is Jason's who is in his late fifties; he was referred by his family physician for unremitting and severe pain in his neck and shoulders following a surgery some years earlier. The surgery was seemingly successful in the early days, but his pain only got worse over time. Prior to the onset of his health problems, he was a very healthy individual engaging in various sports. In college he played hockey and baseball and later he became an avid golfer and angler. He was heavily invested in his physical prowess.

His work history was also quite remarkable. He worked for a newspaper for over two decades, rising to a managerial position, but was unceremoniously dismissed when his job performance suffered because of poor health. He sued his employer and won, but the financial settlement was less than satisfactory. He managed to find another job with much reduced income, but soon after had to go on disability leave due to pain. He was put on disability leave and his income dropped by a full 40%. Jason's family situation was very stable. He was married for 35 years, and the relationship with his wife and two adult daughters was very good. His wife worked in a store as a clerk, which supplemented the family income. Money became an issue for this family. His younger daughter was recently separated and had a daughter with a significant medical problem. Jason felt compelled to help this daughter financially, which was a further drain on his reduced circumstances.

During the initial assessment session, Jason looked sad most of the time, frequently breaking into tears. He was terrified at the prospect of further deterioration in his health. He was depressed and had entertained ideas of suicide from time to time. At the heart of his despair was his very persistent fear of total disability. He assured the therapist that his religious beliefs would prevent him from taking his own life. Nevertheless, the examination of his mental status confirmed that he had slipped into a moderate level of depression.

The rest of the session was devoted to an examination of his willingness to participate in a therapeutic regime that would include medication for pain and depression combined with CBT. He was very motivated to participate and an agreement was reached to offer six sessions of CBT. He responded very well to treatment and over a period of 3 months showed remarkable progress in terms of both pain control and general improvement in his level of functioning. This level of improvement lasted some 6 months and then he had a major setback. He had hoped all along that a surgical intervention was available to "correct" his shoulder problem. He was informed that the decision was not to proceed with the surgery as the risk was too high. This was the beginning of his descent into depression and further medical complication. He started losing his balance and also complained of a loss of memory. He was comprehensively investigated, and the findings were negative. His memory was found to be intact. However, his concentration was compromised.

At the time of writing, he remains sad and very worried about his health. He makes no effort to conceal his disappointment that his "last hope (surgery) for cure" was taken away from him. So far he has shown little motivation to reengage in therapy. This is a story that shows the limitation of CBT, despite initial success, in the face of diminishing circumstances and the loss of hope.

Literature Review

In this section we shall review the literature on meta-analysis of CBT used to treat psychiatric conditions in general and chronic pain in particular. We shall examine application of individual-based and group-based CBT for chronic pain sufferers.

Our focus will be twofold: (1) the lasting effectiveness of CBT and (2) the effectiveness of CBT in addressing some of the issues of social dislocation confronted by chronic pain patients.

It must be acknowledged at the outset that CBT has attained the status of a panacea, and is applied to treat many psychological problems as well as chronic pain (Jackson et al., 2006). In their article, Jackson and colleagues (2006) compared the effectiveness of CBT with that of antidepressants for irritable bowel syndrome, back pain, headache, fibromyalgia, chronic fatigue syndrome, tinnitus, menopausal symptoms, chronic facial pain, noncardiac chest pain, interstitial cystitis, and chronic pelvic pain. For the 11 painful somatic conditions reviewed by Jackson and colleagues (2006), CBT was most consistently demonstrated to be effective. They noted that the quality and quantity of data was varied, ranging from robust to scanty.

Hazlett-Stevens and Craske (2002) also provided a comprehensive review on the effectiveness of brief CBT outcome literature with disorders such as phobias, posttraumatic stress syndrome, anxiety disorders, depression, eating disorders, alcohol use, and pain management. Their overall observation was that, in general, brief CBT was shown to be effective in treating many psychosocial disorders.

In a major meta-analysis of the effectiveness of CBT in treating various psychiatric disorders and chronic pain, Butler and colleagues (2006) demonstrated the effectiveness of CBT in a wide range of disorders such as panic disorder, childhood depression, bulimia, and schizophrenia. They reviewed 16 methodologically rigorous meta-analytic studies and focused on effect sizes that contrasted outcomes for CBT with outcomes for various control groups for each disorder. We report on their findings on two disorders: depression because it is ubiquitous among chromic pain sufferers and chronic pain.

CBT for depression has been subjected to very rigorous scrutiny, but Parker and associates (2003) in their review concluded that this method of intervention was perhaps less effective than its proponents had claimed. However, Butler et al. (2006) noted that Parker et al. (2003) excluded some very high-quality clinical trials that clearly established the superiority of CBT to alternative treatments at follow-up. An earlier meta-analysis conducted by Gloaguen et al. (1998), which Butler et al. (2006) described as the most rigorous meta-analysis on CBT for depression, concluded that CBT was superior to waiting list or placebo controls. The authors noted that because of the popularity of psychodynamic psychotherapy, comparison between this therapy and CBT would be very instructive. However, very few clinical trials have ever been conducted comparing the two.

Elkin and associates (1989) compared the efficacy of CBT, interpersonal psychotherapy, and pharmacotherapy for depression. The outcomes for CBT and interpersonal therapy were almost the same, although CBT fared less well than medication and interpersonal psychotherapy among the more severely depressed patients in this study.

Comparison of CBT with antidepressant medication has shown that the combination of CBT with medication leads to significantly better outcomes with severely depressed patients (Thase et al., 1997). Overall, there is some consensus that CBT as an adjunct has a high degree of efficacy in treating depression. CBT as the treatment of choice has also been demonstrated to be more efficacious than waiting list, attentional controls, and a group of other psychotherapies (Butler et al., 2006).

Chronic Pain and CBT

We begin by reporting on a meta-analysis of 25 trials that tested the efficacy of CBT, which also included behavior therapy and biofeedback with a waiting list and alternative control conditions (Morley et al., 1999). It is noteworthy that Loser (1991) advocated routine treatment with CBT for chronic pain sufferers in view of the fact that other therapies lacked the same level of evidence for efficacy as CBT. Morley and his associates (1999) purported to answer two critical questions in their review: (1) How effective was CBT compared with a WLC in producing changes in a number of variables? (2) How did CBT compare with other treatment or control conditions? This review included individuals, groups, and couples as well as inpatients and outpatients. Diagnosis and the location of pain sites were varied, ranging from rheumatoid arthritis (RA) to mixed chronic pain conditions to low-back pain. Altogether, 76% of the studies in this meta-analysis involved group treatment.

The conclusion with respect to the first question was that CBT was effective in relation to WLC conditions. The results of the meta-analysis clearly established that CBT produced significant changes in a whole host of measures that included pain experience, cognitive coping and appraisal, pain behavior and activity levels, and social role functions.

However, the effectiveness of CBT was measurably lowered across the same range of outcomes when compared with other treatments or conditions. Improvement was confined to pain experience, positive coping, and social role function. A number of critical outcome measures such as healthcare services utilization, drug intake, and change in work role were absent from the studies in their review. Their overall conclusion was that RCTs provided support for the efficacy of CBT in treating a diverse range of chronic pain conditions. There were many methodological issues that had to be addressed in future research.

Ostelo and colleagues (2007) reviewed the efficacy of behavioral treatment (operant, cognitive, and respondent) for CLBP. This review included 21 studies, of which only 7 were considered high quality. Only RCTs were included in this review. The magnitude of effect was assessed by computing a pooled effect size for posttreatment and long-term results for each comparison, for each domain which included overall improvement, specific and generic functional status, return to work, and pain sensitivity using the random effects model.

The findings were complex. For example, in comparison with WLC, behavioral treatment (4 trials and 134 subjects) revealed strong evidence in favor of a combined respondent-cognitive therapy for a medium short-term effect on pain, and moderate evidence (2 trials and 39 subjects) in favor of progressive relaxation for a large positive effect on pain and behavioral outcomes. The authors found limited evidence (6 trials and 210 subjects) that there were no significant differences in short-term or long-term effectiveness when behavioral components were added to the usual treatment for CLBP.

The conclusions the authors drew for this review were that combined respondent-cognitive therapy and progressive relaxation were more effective than WLC for only short-term pain relief. More critically, no differences emerged between behavioral therapies and exercise programs.

It is noteworthy that Van Tulder and associates (1997) had arrived at conclusions similar to those of the preceding review in their analysis of the effectiveness of behavior therapy for CLBP. They identified 11 RCTs, which were deemed "low quality," and 8 of the 11 reported positive and 3 reported negative outcomes. Their conclusion was that the evidence was limited for the effectiveness of behavior therapy for CLBP with good short-term results. There was no evidence that one particular behavior therapy was more effective than the other.

However, Raine and colleagues (2002) had reported positive outcome in their meta-analysis of RCTs of behavior therapy and CBT in treating CLBP. They identified 16 studies of CBT for patients with back pain: 7 in primary care and 9 in secondary care. The outcome was positive in terms of a sustained reduction in pain, disability, and depression. Their meta-analysis of the effectiveness found a moderate positive effect on behavioral outcomes in both the settings. Follow-up in both the settings revealed that the improvements were maintained at 1-year follow-up.

Below we present a selected review of recent studies that used RCTs to test the efficacy of CBT in a diverse group of chronic pain sufferers with different outcomes (Evers et al., 2002; Jensen et al., 2001; Redondo et al., 2004; Turner et al., 2006; Turner-Stokes et al., 2003).

CBT and a Diverse Group of Pain Sufferers

In an unusual Swedish study, the investigators set out to evaluate the outcome of a behavioral medicine (BM) rehabilitation program compared with a TAU control group (CG). The subjects were 214 individuals (97 men and 117 women) suffering from long-term spinal pain. Data were gathered over a period of 4 years and 4 months. The population was drawn from subjects on sick leave identified in a nationwide health insurance scheme. Strict inclusion criteria were established. The purpose of the study was to evaluate the long-term outcome of a BM rehabilitation program. The hypotheses tested were that the treatment conditions should be superior to the control conditions and that full-time BM program should be superior to its main components. Subgroup comparisons were planned in relation to gender.

The treatment conditions were as follows:

(1) The interventions lasted 4 weeks and were conducted in groups of four to eight participants.
(2) All treatments included a physician who examined the patients and was available throughout the intervention for consultations for the patients' medical concerns.

(3) Sessions included two educational sessions on psychological aspects of chronic pain, two on ergonomics, and two on medical aspects of spinal pain.

(4) All treatments included scheduled times for visiting the workplaces, and work managers were invited to participate in the discharge session to decide on a discharge plan.

(5) Six booster sessions were conducted 1 year after the termination of treatment.

Subjects were randomized to one of four conditions:

(1) behavior-oriented physical therapy (PT)
(2) cognitive behavioral therapy (CBT)
(3) BM rehabilitation program consisting of PT + CBT (BM)
(4) a TAU control group (CG)

The outcome variables consisted of sick leave, early retirement, and health-related quality of life (measured using short-form health survey, Short-Form 36 (SF-36)).

Overall, all three treatment conditions yielded similar outcomes compared with the control group. Critically, no significant differences emerged at 18-month follow-up. Further analysis yielded some interesting findings in that a number of differences emerged regarding early retirement and health-related quality of life related to interventions in comparison with CG. Curiously, the positive effects of interventions were confined to females. No significant differences were found for the males on SF-36. The authors concluded that the results revealed gender differences in the outcome of the treatment and the components of the BM program were as effective as the whole program.

This finding was contrary to the hypothesis and the authors noted that from a clinical point of view it was critical to ascertain what might have been lacking or what could be improved in the rehabilitation programs with regard to their ability to facilitate their return to work. Basically, with the exception of some gender differences, this study failed to establish the superiority of CBT to standard treatment in this particular rehabilitation program. A number of plausible causes were offered to explain the null findings of this study. The reasons offered included the use of a population-based sample, the length of sick leave (4 months on average) of the subjects, which probably did not provide enough time for effective intervention, sampling bias such as women in the PT or CBT conditions were just as likely to seek treatment, but less likely to be awarded, and an earlier retirement than that of participants in the other conditions. Obviously, this study needs replication with an improved methodology.

Our next study also failed to demonstrate the efficacy or superiority of CBT to a physical exercise–based strategy (PE) in the treatment of a group of female patients with fibromyalgia (Rodendo et al., 2004). This was a prospective long-term randomized controlled study that investigated the respective merit of the two treatment groups. Patients who met the criteria of fibromyalgia were randomly assigned to the CBT group ($n = 21$) and to the PE group ($n = 19$).

The outcome measures included physical activity, aerobic capacity, Fibromyalgia Impact Questionnaire (FIQ), Short-Form 36 (SF-36), Beck Anxiety and Depression Inventory, Chronic Pain Self-Efficacy Scale, and Chronic Pain Coping Inventory. The PE group at the end of the 8-week treatment showed significant improvement in most items and total score on the FIQ. On the SF-36, only the bodily pain domain showed a significant improvement. No differences were found on the psychological measures. However, physical activity showed significant improvement. At 6-month follow-up most of the clinical variables had returned to the baseline, and at 1-year follow-up all the improvements basically returned to the baseline.

The results were very similar for the CBT group. Initially, significant improvements were noted on a number of measures such as the utilization of strategies and relaxation to cope with pain. However, no significant improvement was noted on the psychological variables. Only physical activity of the vertebral column showed moderate improvement after treatment. At 6-month follow-up all the clinical variables on the FIQ returned to baseline values, although significant improvements were noted on the physical function and general health domains on the SF-36. At 1-year follow-up all the clinical variables had returned to the baseline values. Analgesic intake, in fact, showed a rise at this point. Between-group comparison at the 1-year follow-up did not reveal any statistical differences on any of the clinical variables or consumption of medication.

The authors noted that one of the most significant findings of their study was that the beneficial effects of the two interventions disappeared over time. Only physical fitness in the PE group was better at follow-up. The authors concluded that the physical improvement in patients with fibromyalgia did not necessarily correlate with an improvement in the clinical manifestations of the disease. The most telling aspect of this study was that PE failed to maintain the same improvement in the physical domain as CBT in the psychological domain. Both therapies were ineffective after 1 year of termination. No satisfactory explanation was offered for these findings.

The next study in this section is altogether more optimistic, and indeed takes CBT research into a relatively new domain (Turner et al., 2006). This study was unique for the reason that it tested the efficacy of CBT as a brief as well as a long-term therapy in the treatment of patients with temporomandibular disorder (TMD) and clearly specified primary and secondary outcomes, process variables, and the clinical significance criterion for pain. Subjects were randomly assigned to either four sessions of CBT ($n = 79$) or an education/attention control condition ($n = 79$). Inclusion criteria were as follows: (1) age 18 or older; (2) a confirmed diagnosis of TMD made by an oral medicine specialist; (3) residence within a 2-h drive from the TMD clinic; (4) facial pain of 3 months' duration; (5) carefully defined categories of facial pain–related disability; and (6) the ability to communicate in English.

The outcome was measured in terms of interference with activities and pain intensity, limitations related to the use of jaw, and depression. The authors also created another category of outcome that they termed as process measure, which assessed dimensions such as pain beliefs and coping with pain, and also the subject's knowledge about their medical condition and the credibility of the treatment(s) they were to receive. The helpfulness of treatment was assessed at the point of termination. Standardized instruments were used for all the outcome measures.

The results were unequivocal in demonstrating the superiority of CBT over the control condition. The CBT intervention compared with the control condition produced statistically and clinically significant improvement in the domain of activity interference, pain, depression, and jaw function over the following year. With regard to process measures, the CBT patients also showed significant changes in their pain-related beliefs that are known to contribute to pain and disability. Improvement was also evident during the year after treatment in that there was a greater decrease in the pain belief that they were disabled and that their pain signaled harm; also, there was an increase in the perceived ability to control pain and related problems. The authors concluded that their findings supported the cognitive behavioral model of chronic pain. The outcome of this study established a clear rationale for implementation of brief CBT alongside medical intervention in the treatment of chronic pain, and specific ingredients of CBT were recognized as responsible for the improvements.

In a recent article Turner and colleagues (2007) tested key mediators such as pain coping, catastrophizing, self-efficacy, and pain beliefs that were critical to establishing the mechanisms of CBT pain management protocols. This study was a further analysis of the data of their previous study reported earlier. One central finding was that in individual mediator analysis, change in perceived control was the mediator that explained the greatest proportion of the total treatment effect on each outcome. Furthermore, the effects of CBT did not vary much according to the patient's baseline, suggesting that all patients may potentially benefit from CBT. Commenting on this article in an editorial in the journal *Pain*, Morley and Keefe (2007) observed that this was the very first study to conduct such mediational analysis in the context of an RCT of CBT for pain management. They further noted that such a rigorous approach represented a methodological improvement over prior studies in that the treatment protocols for CBT and the control conditions were standardized, the outcome measures state of the art, and the evaluations conducted at specified time points.

Our next study involves the application of customized CBT for patients with relatively early RA (Evers et al., 2002). A total of 112 patients met the criteria for a psychosocial risk profile in comparison with patients not at risk such as in terms of significantly higher levels of negative mood and anxiety, greater helplessness and less acceptance, more passive coping with pain, and lower levels of social functioning for perceived support and the social network. Sixty-four patients agreed to participate in the study.

The 64 patients were randomly assigned to one of two conditions: standard treatment for RA and CBT. The CBT condition consisted of individual treatment with two of four possible treatment modules that targeted the most frequently experienced problems experienced by RA patients: pain and functional disability, fatigue, negative mood, and social relationships. The outcome measures consisted of physical and psychosocial functioning.

Significant improvements on physical, psychological, and social functioning were reported by the CBT completers when compared with the controls. Effect sizes of the primary outcome measures with significant effects revealed overall medium effects for the CBT condition at posttreatment and at follow-up. The authors concluded that customized CBT for patients with early RA, a tailor-made therapy offered to individuals at psychosocial risk, had significant beneficial effects on the primary outcomes of physical, psychological, and social functioning.

The results showed overall benefits of CBT on physical, psychological, and social functioning. Specifically, fatigue and depression were significantly reduced at posttreatment and at 6-month follow-up. Furthermore, helplessness decreased and active coping increased both at posttreatment and at 6-month follow-up. The CBT group also showed a greater level of compliance with medication than the control condition.

The final study in this section compared group CBT with an individual therapy for treating a rather diverse group of chronic pain sufferers (Turner-Stokes et al., 2003). Participants had to have pain of 6 months' duration; be impervious to medical treatment; and be 18 years and older. A total of 126 subjects were randomly assigned to two treatment groups: group CBT and an individual therapy condition. CBT groups consisted of eight to ten patients and they attended sessions for one full afternoon a week for 8 weeks. In addition to CBT, patients also received physiotherapy, occupational therapy, and medical treatment. They were also taught relaxation and cognitive coping strategies.

The individual program included a 1-h session every other week and the patients received the same information as the CBT group. Treatment was delivered by a psychologist. Findings of physiotherapy assessment determined the physical activity and exercise program. All advice was tailored to the individual needs.

The outcome measures were obtained using standardized instruments and included interference of pain with daily activities and patient's sense of control over pain and depression. In addition, state and trait anxiety, analgesic medication consumption, and antiinflammatory drugs consumed over a week, physical and social activity inside and outside the home, and pain severity were also measured.

Of the 126 subjects who started the program, 113 completed (66 in the group and 47 in the individual program). No differences emerged between the two treatment conditions either at the point of termination or at 6-month and 12-month follow-ups. Persons who received individual therapy demonstrated a lesser tendency to relapse after the treatment. In conclusion, the two programs were found equally efficacious for pain management in adults with chronic pain.

Summary

This brief and selected review of meta-analysis produced rather conflicting results in terms of the efficacy of CBT to treat chronic pain. Morley et al.'s (1999) report was encouraging to the extent that CBT was clearly superior to waiting list and other control conditions, albeit, less so. Raine and colleagues (2002) also reported a positive outcome of CBT with CLBP both at the point of termination and at

1-year follow-up. The finding of the Cochrane Review (Ostelo et al., 2007) was less sanguine. Compared with WLCs, behavioral interventions were beneficial in the short run, but compared with exercise programs, behavioral treatments yielded the same level of efficacy. One shortcoming of the Cochrane Review was the failure to conduct a cost-effectiveness analysis. Given that the two conditions of treatment were more or less equivalent, such an analysis could have given some direction in terms of choice of therapy in terms of cost of treatment.

In the preceding section we reviewed several reports that investigated the efficacy of CBT in treating specific pain disorders, namely, fibromyalgia, spinal pain, temporomandibular joint pain, RA, and a more general mix of chronic pain conditions. The first two studies reported no measurable benefits of CBT, whereas the latter two studies not only reported significant benefits, but were also noteworthy for their innovative design that led to considerable refinement of CBT. Our last study demonstrated that individual treatment and group-based CBT had the same efficacy. One question we posed at the beginning of this review was if the studies involving CBT reported on social functioning of their subjects. All the studies had included some measure to determine the impact of CBT on social functions. The instruments were varied, but in broad and general terms; collectively, the studies reported significant improvement in social functions such as general functional status, social activities, and activities of daily living.

At least, on the basis of this selected review on the efficacy of CBT in treating either general chronic pain conditions or specific pain disorders, the outcome is mixed. On the contrary, CBT is unquestionably superior to no-treatment conditions. In comparison with other treatments, CBT is either less effective or equally effective.

Headache and CBT

Now we provide a selected overview of the more recent literature assessing the efficacy of CBT in treating chronic head pain. Holroyd and Penzien (1994) provided a comprehensive and sweeping review of the treatment literature on migraine and tension headaches. This included relaxation training, biofeedback, CBT, which they described as stress management, and minimal-contact treatment format, which included up to four monthly sessions of therapy.

They reviewed five outcome studies of CBT related to tension-type headaches and noted that the usefulness of CBT was evident in all of them. Furthermore, CBT probably added to the effectiveness of biofeedback and relaxation training for certain subgroups of headache sufferers. They postulated that patients most likely to benefit from CBT as an adjunct to relaxation therapy could be the patients for whom psychological problems such as chronic daily stress, depression, and adjustment problems aggravated or interfered with skills derived from relaxation or biofeedback therapy.

Their conclusion regarding migraine was that no evidence was available to suggest that CBT added significantly to the effectiveness of relaxation or biofeedback.

One reason for the lack of effectiveness of CBT was attributed to the fact that CBT was specifically developed for treating tension-type headaches. They postulated that CBT would require modification to be more conducive to treat migraine. They concluded that CBT added little to the treatment and management of migraine.

Goslin and associates (1999) analyzed 39 prospective and randomized trials to determine the effectiveness of behavioral treatments for migraine. Behavioral interventions that included relaxation, EMG biofeedback, and CBT yielded 32–49% reduction in migraine versus 5% reduction for no-treatment control. The behavioral therapies were all statistically more effective than WLC. A more recent review reported that behavioral treatments including relaxation, biofeedback, and CBT yielded a 35–55% reduction in migraine and tension headaches, with effects lasting up to 7 years, the longest reported follow-up (Raines et al., 2005).

Penzien and colleagues (2002) also noted that the evidence for drug and nondrug treatments for headaches indicated that the level of headache reduction with behavioral interventions may rival those obtained with widely used pharmacological therapies in representative patient samples. They cautioned, however, that systematic comparison had just begun and should await further corroboration (Penzien et al., 2002). Andrasik (2004), however, cautioned that despite three decades of research affirming the effectiveness of behavioral therapies for headaches, the literature base was much less extensive for chronic and refractory headaches.

Our final review investigated 14 studies that examined the cognitive behavioral model in treating chronic headache and low-back pain (Jaklean and Basler, 2000). Inclusion criteria for the meta-analysis were as follows: prospective controlled design with randomized assignment of patients, cognitive behavioral treatment, measurement of cognitive variables pretreatment and posttreatment, report means and standard deviations for experimental and control conditions, and a minimum sample size of five for each treatment group.

For the headache patients cognitive variables showed a strong effect size ($d+ = 0.88$), in contrast to the low-back subjects who showed a weak effect size ($d+ = 0.30$). The findings established that CBT resulted in an improvement in pain-related condition, but the magnitude of change depended on the pain diagnosis. The authors concluded that the cognitive behavioral model was supported by their findings.

Summary

In broad terms evidence suggests that CBT in combination with other behavioral interventions is superior to waiting list in treating head pain. However, McCrory and colleagues (2001) warned that although behavioral treatments for tension-type headaches have consistently yielded positive outcome, the collection of trials and the results of meta-analysis provided little guidance for choosing among the treatments (relaxation training, CBT with relaxation training and without, EMG biofeedback combined with relaxation and without). They noted that the summary effect size estimates made various categories of behavior therapy statistically indistinguishable. The effectiveness of CBT and other behavioral interventions for the treatment of migraine remains an open question.

Conclusion

This chapter presented a selected review of the literature on the effectiveness of CBT in treating chronic pain conditions. The evidence, though mixed, points to the general usefulness of CBT in treating chronic pain, often in conjunction with other psychological and pharmacological therapies. Nevertheless, research has consistently shown that when compared with no-treatment/control conditions, CBT has been demonstrated to be effective in significantly reducing pain severity, affective distress, and disability following the intervention up to 6 months posttreatment. Research urges further refinement of CBT to augment the cognitive behavioral model of pain that underlies this therapy. Furthermore, Andrasik (2004) observed that behavioral interventions have been quite effective for uncomplicated types of headaches and proposed that the role of environmental and familial factors in influencing chronic headaches required further research. Perhaps the same observation can be made for other chronic pain conditions. As of now, it would be an overestimation of the effectiveness of CBT to regard it as a panacea for treating chronic pain conditions.

Beyond the superiority of CBT to WLC conditions, evidence for the effectiveness of CBT for chronic pain conditions assumes a certain level of complexity. The Cochrane Review (Ostelo et al., 2007) reported earlier asserted the time-limited value of CBT. Other studies failed to show the superiority of CBT over other behavioral and physical interventions. Another point of note is that group-based and individual-based CBT seem to yield similar outcomes. This would suggest that group-based CBT would be economically more viable simply because this approach would treat a larger number of patients.

To return for a moment to our patients described at the outset, it remains unclear as to the criteria for patient selection for CBT. One patient with headache, a high-functioning teacher, benefited greatly, and another patient with a complicated clinical picture, after initial success, relapsed, thus supporting the Cochrane Review conclusion about the short-term nature of the benefit of CBT. The selection criteria for CBT as the treatment of choice require further research. Holroyd and Penzien (1994), however, noted that chronic pain patients with marked psychological problems related to daily stress, depression, and adjustment problems were most likely to benefit from CBT. Nevertheless, based on the current state of knowledge, the idea of "one treatment fits all" may not apply to CBT for treating all chronic pain sufferers.

References

Andrasik, F. (2004) Behavioral treatment approaches to chronic headache. Neurol. Sci., 24(Suppl. 2): s80–s85.

Butler, A., Chapman, J., Forman, E., and Beck, A. (2006) The empirical status of cognitive-behavioral therapy: a review of meta-analysis. Clin. Psychol. Rev., 26: 17–31.

Evers, A., Kraaimatt, F., van Riel, P., and de Jong, A. (2002) Tailored cognitive-behavioral therapy in early rheumatoid arthritis: a randomized controlled trial. Pain, 100: 141–153.

Elkin, I., Shea, M., Watkins, S., et al. (1989) National Institute of Mental Health Treatment of Depression Collaborative Research Program: general effectiveness of treatments. Arch. Gen. Psychiatry, 46: 971–982.

Gloaguen, V., Cottraux, J., Cucherat, M., and Blackburn, I. (1998) A meta-analysis of the effects of cognitive therapy in depressed patients. J. Affect. Disord., 49: 59–72.

Goslin, R., Gray, R., McCrory, D., et al. (1999) Behavioral and physical treatments for migraine headaches. Technical Review 2.2. Prepared for the Agency for Health Care Policy and Research (Contract no. 290-94-2025).

Hazlett-Stevens, H. and Craske, M. (2002) Brief cognitive behavioral therapy: definition and scientific foundation. In: Bond, F. and Dryden, W. (Eds.) Handbook of Brief Cognitive Behavior Therapy. John Wiley and Sons. London.

Holroyd, K. and Penzien, D. (1994) Psychosocial interventions in the management of recurrent headache disorders. Behav. Med., 20: 53–68.

Holzman, A., Turk. D., and Kerns, R. (1986) The cognitive-behavioral approach to management of chronic pain. In: A. Holzman and D. Turk (Eds.) Pain Management: A Handbook of Psychological Approaches (pp. 31–50). Elmsford, NY, Pergamon Press.

Jackson, J., O'Malley, P., and Kroenke, K. (2006) Antidepressants and cognitive behavioral therapy for symptom syndromes. CNS Spectr., 11: 212–222.

Jaklean, C. and Basler, H. (2000) Change in cognition in psychological pain therapy: a meta-analysis of the cognitive behavioral model. Zeitschrift fur Klinische Psychol. Psychother., 29: 127–139.

Jensen, I., Bergstrom, G., Ljungquist, T., Bodin, L., and Nygren, A. (2001) A randomized controlled component analysis of a behavioral medicine rehabilitation program for chronic spinal pain: are the effects dependent on gender? Pain, 91: 65–78.

Loser, J. (1991) The role of chronic pain clinics in managing back pain. In: Frymoyer, J. (Ed.) The Adult Spine: Principles and Practice (pp. 221–229). New York, Raven Press.

McCrory, D., Penzien, D., Hasselblad, V., and Gray, R. (2001) Evidence report: behavioral and physical treatments for tension type and cervicogenic headache. Product no. 2085.

Morley, S., Eccleston, C., and Williams, A. (1999) Systemic review and meta-analysis of randomized controlled trials of cognitive behavior therapy and behavior therapy for chronic pain in adults, excluding headache. Pain, 80: 1–13.

Morley, S. and Keefe, F. (2007) Getting a handle on process and change in CBT for chronic pain. Pain, 127: 197–198.

Ostelo, M., van Tulder, M., Vlaeyen, J., et al. (2007) Behavioral treatment for chronic low-back pain. Cochrane Database Syst. Rev., Issue 1.

Parker, G., Roy, K., and Eyers, K. (2003) Cognitive behavior therapy for depression? Choose horses for courses. Am. J. Psychiatry, 160: 825–834.

Penzien, D., Rains, J., and Andrasik, F. (2002) Behavioral management of recurrent headache: three decades of experience and empiricism. Appl. Psychophysiol. Biofeedback, 27: 163–181.

Raine, R., Haines, A., Sensky, T., et al. (2002) Systematic review of mental health interventions for patients with common somatic symptoms: can research evidence from secondary care be extrapolated to primary care? BMJ, 325: 1082–1097.

Raines, J., Penzien, D., McCrory, D., and Gray, R. (2005) Behavioral headache treatment: history, review of the empirical literature, and methodological critique. Headache, 45(Suppl. 2): s92–s109.

Redondo, J., Justo, C., Moraleda, F., et al. (2004) Long-term efficacy of therapy with patients with fibromyalgia: a physical exercise-based program and a cognitive behavioral approach. Arthritis Rheum., 51: 184–192.

Thase, E., Greenhouse, J., Frank, E., et al. (1997) Treatment of major depression with psychotherapy or psychotherapy-pharmacotherapy combinations. Arch. Gen. Psychiatry, 54: 1009–1015.

Turk, D. (2002) A cognitive-behavioral perspective on treatment of chronic pain patients. In: D. Turk and R. Gatchell (Eds.) Psychological Approaches to Pain Management: A Practitioner's Handbook, 2nd edn (pp. 138–158). New York, Guilford Press.

Turk, D. and Gatchell, R. (2002) Psychological Approaches to Pain Management. New York, Guilford Press.

Turk, D., Meichenbaum, D., and Genest, M. (1983) Pain and Behavioral Medicine: A Cognitive-Behavioral Perspective. New York, Guilford Press.

Turner, J., Holtzman, S., and Manel, S. (2007) Mediators, moderators, and predictors of therapeutic change in cognitive-behavioral therapy for chronic pain. Pain, 127: 276–286.

Turner, J., Manel, L., and Aaron, L. (2006) Short and long-term efficacy of brief cognitive behavioral therapy for patients with chronic temporomandibular disorder pain: a randomized controlled trial. Pain, 121: 181–194.

Turner-Stokes, L., Erkeller-Yuksel, F., Miles, A., et al. (2003) Outpatient cognitive behavioral pain management programs: a randomized comparison of a group-based multi-disciplinary versus an individual therapy model. Arch. Phys. Med. Rehabil., 84: 781–788.

Van Tulder, M., Koes, B., and Bouter, L. (1997) Conservative treatment of acute and chronic non-specific low-back pain: a systematic review of randomized controlled trials of the most common interventions. Spine, 22: 2128–2156.

Chapter 9
Group Therapy

Group therapy as a method of intervention has been in wide use in treating chronic pain. As was evident in the previous chapter, CBT-based group therapy has come under much scrutiny, and as such, with some minor exception, we are excluding this body of literature from this review. This chapter will provide an overview of group therapy followed by group therapy in relation to mixed pain groups, headache, and fibromyalgia. We shall also present a brief review of group therapy and depression literature because depression or depressive symptoms are all too common among the chronic pain sufferers. Only relatively recent literature, with some minor exceptions, is included in this review.

Group Therapy and Medical Illness

In a comprehensive review of the outcome literature on group therapy for the medically ill, Vamos (2006) noted that group psychotherapy, providing an environment to share experience, has obvious advantages and has been frequently used in either a supportive or a CBT format. Incidentally, this review provides an extensive review of group CBT literature for the treatment of the medically ill.

Vamos' (2006) review of the outcome of group therapy casts a very wide net and includes cancer (Cain et al., 1986), HIV (Goodwin et al., 2001; Kelly et al., 1993; Markowitz, et al., 2000), renal transplant (Baines et al., 2004), chronic obstructive airways disease (DeGoody and de Godoy, 2003), and heart disease (Rahe et al., 1979). Vamos' conclusion of the current state of psychotherapy for the medically ill is less than optimistic. She noted that there was an overall paucity of well-designed studies that unambiguously showed psychotherapy as an effective treatment in the medically ill. Her central concern was that a clear conceptual thread recognizing the long-term and diverse experience of patients with medical illness and relating this to the part psychotherapy should play was lacking.

A meta-analysis of 23 outcome studies that directly compared the effectiveness of individual and group therapy concluded that no differences were found in the outcome (McRoberts et al., 1998). The meta-analysis included 23 outcome studies that directly compared individual with group interventions. They were discouraged by the fact that only 23 studies could be included in their analysis after nearly

R. Roy, *Psychosocial Interventions for Chronic Pain*,
DOI: 10.1007/978-0-387-76296-8_9 © Springer Science+Business Media, LLC 2008

50 years of investigation of psychotherapy outcome research. One of the limitations of this study, the authors noted, was that only 12% of the planned analysis in this meta-analysis lacked sufficient sample size to determine differential effectiveness, and 92% of the variables produced nonsignificant *t* tests with low power. They ended on an optimistic note stating that much of the information lacking in the literature, such as on client, therapist, group, methodological and treatment variables, could be easily obtained in the managed care environment. This study found that group therapy could be used as an efficacious cost-effective alternative to individual therapy.

Group Therapy and Depression

We report on two meta-analytic reviews of group therapy and depression. Our reason for this brief incursion into this body of literature is the wide prevalence of depression and depressive symptoms in the chronic pain population. Conversely, somatic symptoms, including pain, are equally observable in the depressed patients. There are additional findings that may be of relevance to the chronic pain population.

Engels and Vermey (1997) reported on a meta-analysis of 17 studies on the efficacy of psychological treatments for depression in the elderly. These 17 studies used 28 psychotherapeutic treatments on 732 depressed seniors. The overall result showed that on average the treated patient was 74% better off than the patients in control conditions. Cognitive therapy and behavior therapy were the most successful treatments. Another critical finding was the superiority of individual therapy over group therapy. Treatment was more successful in patients with the diagnosis of major depression or depression than in patients with mixed diagnosis. The treatment was equally successful with mild and severe depression. Patients with multiple problems were found to be problematic. The younger elderly seemed to benefit more from therapy than their older counterparts.

Cognitive and behavior therapies yielded better outcome than CBT. These therapies were also superior to relaxation therapy, structured reminiscent training, physical training, anger expression, and music therapy. Placebo treatments, mostly attention placebos, produced considerable therapeutic effects.

McDermut and associates (2001) conducted a meta-analysis of 48 research reports on the efficacy of group therapy for depression. Fifteen of these studies compared treated subjects with untreated controls. The types of therapy employed in these studies included behavioral, cognitive, CBT, psychodynamic–interpersonal, social support, nondirective attention-control, and "others."

Of the 48 studies, 43 studies concluded that group psychotherapy was effective in reducing depressive symptoms following therapy. Only 3 of 46 studies failed to establish any beneficiary outcome of group therapy. The meta-analysis established that the on average the treated participant was 84.7% better off than the untreated participants.

On comparing group therapy with individual therapy, based on effect sizes, five studies favored individual therapy over group therapy and four studies favored group therapy over individual therapy. CBT was found to be only "slightly" superior to psychodynamic psychotherapy.

The authors' overall conclusion, however, was that based on meta-analysis there was no evidence that individual therapy was superior to group intervention. Nevertheless, group therapy was more cost-effective and could serve as a first intervention in a stepped-up program. The mere presence of other individuals in the therapy room could produce numerous curative factors. The subjects in their meta-analysis were, at best, moderately depressed.

Summary

The points worth noting from these two studies are as follows:

(1) Behavioral therapies are superior to other forms of psychotherapy.
(2) The first study involving elderly subjects reported individual therapy as superior to group therapy. Our second study provided more convincing data for greater efficacy of group therapy. Both studies, however, were tentative in terms of superiority of group therapy over individual therapy. Cost-effectiveness of group therapy was proffered as a consideration. However, neither study presented any cost-effectiveness-related data.
(3) Both studies reported success with "uncomplicated" depression and even severe depression, as in the first study, and had questions about the efficacy of group therapy when depression coexisted with other medical conditions. In the second study, only moderately depressed individuals were represented. This last finding may have some bearing on the treatment of chronic pain sufferers where the clinical picture is often complicated, and pain and depression are commonly encountered in this population.

Group Social Support Interventions

Social support is often a casualty of chronic illness and pain. Roy (2007) noted that among the chronic pain population, there is a marked decrease in informal and semiformal support while the involvement with formal systems such as hospitals and WCB and insurance companies seems to rise. We begin this section with a brief examination of social support interventions for a mixed group of medically ill patients. In a recent review of literature Hogan and colleagues (2002) observed that despite a massive amount of empirical support showing the benefits of social support, there was surprisingly little hard evidence about how and how well social support interventions worked.

Group interventions reviewed by Hogan and associates (2002) included support through (1) social support intervention for family and/or friends, (2) peer support groups, (3) support groups as means for providing social support, and (4) social support skills training. These four types of group interventions were used with problems of overweight, alcoholism, drug addiction, breast cancer, multiple sclerosis, bulimia, rheumatoid arthritis, and psychiatric problems. Overall, the results were encouraging. A summary of the results indicated that social support interventions were generally successful.

Eight studies that reviewed groups involving family/friends showed positive outcome for social support intervention. Results were stable over time. Most of the interventions were behaviorally oriented. In five of the six studies involving a peer or self-help group, the outcome was positive, and an improvement in general well-being or specific symptomatology was reported. The authors cautioned that the results must be interpreted with caution because not one study in this group employed a randomized control group design. In the third category of support groups as a means of social support, five studies targeted psychiatric populations. Skills training consistently improved assertion and social functioning. In the final category of group interventions that combined provisions of support with skills training, only one such study was located. This study involved patients with HIV who had recently lost a friend. The results showed that this intervention was successful in reducing grief.

In terms of all types of social support interventions, the authors concluded that of the 100 studies reviewed, 39 reported that supportive interventions were superior to no-treatment or standard care controls, 12 reported that interventions were superior or equivalent to alternate, 22 suggested partial benefits of social support interventions, and 17 reported no benefits. In eight studies there were no controls and comparison was not possible. In sum, 83% of the studies reported some benefit.

The next study is probably the most comprehensive and systematic review of social support interventions with type 2 diabetes (Van Dam et al., 2005). The literature search identified 69 trials with acceptable methodological designs: RCT or quasi-experimental. Another 63 studies were excluded as they involved type 1 diabetes. This left six studies for inclusion in this review.

This review, while confirming the overall benefits of social support intervention, failed to clarify which aspects of social support, and what mechanisms behind it, were most effective for promoting self-management and outcomes of care for persons with type 2 diabetes. One example of such a complication was the negative effect of social support on spousal participation in weight loss education groups for obese men with type 2 diabetes. Spousal support in that situation was experienced as nagging or harassment, and probably acted negatively on dietary adherence. On the contrary, social support from peers and fellow patients, both in groups, peer group sessions, telephone peer contacts, or Internet-based communication could contribute to lifestyle adjustments and outcomes of care. Although patient group consultations with physicians, peer groups, and peer counselors had positive outcome for certain patients, there were no effects on diabetes control for family and friend participation in diabetes education groups, or from social support groups for older male patients. The authors carefully concluded that their review provided support for the hypothesis that specific social support interventions influenced self-care and diabetes outcome.

Our final report is that of a wide-ranging review of the literature on social support interventions for patients with rheumatoid arthritis (RA) (Lanza and Revenson, 1993). These authors made a critical observation by noting that social support was an integral component of any kind of group therapy. They noted that counseling and group therapy interventions involved a discussion of salient arthritis issues, and their underlying goal of creating an atmosphere of mutual support in which to openly discuss emotional and practical issues meant including a variety of studies in their review even though the stated purpose of some of these interventions may not have explicitly made any reference to social support.

In describing multimodal interventions, these authors reported two studies. One compared a mutual support group and stress management and a no-treatment control group. The other compared efficacy of CBT, social support, social support only, and a no-treatment condition. The first study failed to establish significant differences between the two groups and concluded that mutual support group and stress management may not help RA patients, and suggested more powerful interventions for patients with long-term disease. The other study reported reduction in anxiety in both treatment groups, although all three conditions showed increased disease activity and depression. In a 6-month follow-up, only the CBT group maintained its improvement. All in all, social support intervention as part of a multitreatment model failed to produce the desired effect.

Their conclusions, based on a variety of support interventions that included family and friends, were complex and less than optimistic. First, an assumption that all individuals were somehow lacking in social support may not be correct. Second, that more support was necessarily better. The fact was that negative consequences of support were rarely taken into account. Individual patients varied enormously in their response to group interventions by reacting with fear and trepidation to the problems of their fellow patients. Patients in the advance stage of disease may contribute to serious anxiety and foreboding in some patients. Finally, all well-intended support efforts may not be perceived as such by the recipients. For example, family involvement in support therapy may produce paradoxical results whereby patients may feel more controlled by specific family members. The authors urged that implementation of interventions that were theory driven was based on an enhanced understanding of the support process, and a clear understanding of the mechanisms of support.

Support for the views of the abovementioned authors can be found in a very concise article on physiological processes underlying support and its impact on health (Uchino et al., 1999). They noted that there was a great deal of empirical literature to show a clear relationship between the level of support and risk for a variety of diseases such as cardiovascular, cancer, and infectious diseases. However, in agreement with Lanza and Revenson (1993), Uchino and colleagues (1999) were equally puzzled about the underlying process that might enable social support to act as a buffer. Literature did not shed much light on that question. Nevertheless, they strongly recommended that it may be worthwhile to incorporate social support interventions in the prevention and treatment of physical health problems.

Summary

First and foremost, research reports on the efficacy of social support interventions with chronic pain sufferers are noteworthy by their virtual absence. Our last review with RA only succeeded in adding further complications to the question of effectiveness, although social support interventions were strongly recommended with that population.

Despite somewhat mixed results in so far as the efficacy of social support intervention is concerned, its usefulness, albeit somewhat constrained, was reported in relation to both depression and diabetes. Our last two reviews raised serious theoretical questions related to mechanisms and physiological processes that may explain the curative or ameliorative process of social support interventions. Although at a common sense level as well as empirically the benefits of social support with physically ill patients including chronic pain sufferers are well documented (Roy, 2001), the extent of the implementation of therapy associated with social support for chronic pain sufferers remains questionable.

Group Therapy and Mixed Pain

A number of studies have reported on the effectiveness of group therapy of various kinds in treating groups of chronic pain sufferers with differing pain sites and diagnosis. Group therapy, in general as well as specific terms, was sometimes found to be effective in dealing with specific problems. For example, in a comprehensive multidisciplinary treatment program comprising a whole range of interventions that ranged from heat treatment to social work, group therapy was found to be effective with patients who showed some signs of confusion and vigor, although in the overall scheme of treatment effectiveness, group therapy was not significant (Kleinke, 1987).

Another article reported using group therapy sessions for stress management and pain-coping skills and another group format to teach the anatomy and physiology of pain, medications, proper body mechanisms, activities of daily living, and behavior change principles (Dolce et al., 1986). Subjects were 63 chronic pain patients who were involved in a multidisciplinary pain treatment program. Unfortunately, this study, unlike, the previous, did not report separately on the effectiveness of individual treatment methods. We shall discuss these two reports in detail in the next chapter, which examines the efficacy of multidisciplinary pain management and treatment programs.

Gamsa and associates (1985) reported on the use of structured group therapy sessions in treating chronic pain sufferers. This was not an empirical study. The group format was open-ended. In the course of 10 weeks, 3 males and 7 females participated in group therapy. The purpose of the group was mutual support and enhancement of activity levels and self-confidence. Patients were found to be very supportive of each other. Psychological conflicts were acknowledged and feelings of sadness and anger were freely expressed. Based on the observation, the authors concluded that group sessions were beneficial despite some initial resistance particularly in relation to disclosure of psychological conflicts. They recommended incorporation of group therapy in any multidisciplinary pain treatment program.

Weir and colleagues (1988) also reported their experience of successful group therapy program, which involved 12 patients. The group was heterogeneous in their demographics and diagnosis. The purpose was to provide behavioral and cognitive techniques for pain control and involvement of spouse or significant others to enhance therapeutic effects. The groups were closed and met for 5 weeks for two 2-h sessions. Each session was preplanned. Major themes that emerged during the sessions were loss and grieving, helplessness, isolation, and anger and depression. The majority of the participants moved through identifiable stages of attitude and behavior change, and over time, the group developed competence in managing their responses to pain. Overall, the group experience was deemed as useful for the patients.

It must be acknowledged that the previous two articles discussed above were strictly clinical, devoid of any empirical support for their report of successful outcome and must be judged as such. The following two reports, however, are empirically derived, and for this reason we present them in some detail (Boyle and Ciccone, 1994; Dahl and Fallstrom, 1989).

Dahl and Fallstrom (1989) reported on the effectiveness of a behavior group therapy with a heterogeneous group of chronic pain sufferers. Therapy involved relaxation training, contingency management of pain behavior, and social skills training. Nine men and fifteen women participated in this study; they were divided into three groups of eight each. An AB design entailing a 2-week baseline, an 8-week intervention (2/6 hours session/week), and a 6-month follow-up was implemented. The goal of the treatment was to identify specific pain-related behaviors and to modify these learned patterns. A broad range of instruments were used to measure pain-related behaviors before, during, and after treatment.

The results, based on t tests, showed significant changes from baseline to follow-up—reduction in the intake of pain medication, average number of rests per day, and pain intensity. The authors concluded that behaviorally oriented group intervention was capable of reducing pain symptoms and enhancing healthy behaviors. However, they cautioned that the absence of a control group prevented the control of spontaneous progression of the pain behaviors measured.

Finally, we report a study that investigated the effects of relaxation versus relaxation combined with rational emotive therapy on mood and pain (Boyle and Ciccone, 1994). Thirty-four chronic pain patients were assigned to three groups. Mean age of the sample was 61.06 years (SD = 12.9 years). They were taught progressive muscle relaxation and guided imagery techniques. Training also included autogenic training and controlled breathing techniques. Treatment with relaxation and rational emotive therapy was rooted in the stress inoculation approach, which is partly derived from rational emotive therapy. The treatment consisted of once-weekly 90-minute sessions over 5 consecutive weeks. There were no drop-outs from either treatment condition. A number of instruments were used to measure the improvement in pain levels and mood.

This was a quasi-experimental design. The results were equivocal at best. Relaxation alone failed to decrease negative mood states significantly. Relaxation with rational emotive therapy alone decreased negative affectivity, increased arousal and energy level, and increased friendliness. On most of the subscales on the psychometric outcome measures (POMS), scores of the relaxation therapy alone increased marginally. This was contrary to prediction.

The authors concluded that despite the fact that relaxation with rational emotive therapy had little impact on the alleviation of pain, this method had some positive effects on patients' emotions and feelings, and by inference, on their level of functioning. Rational emotive therapy with relaxation was seen as a justifiable undertaking in treating older chronic pain sufferers.

Summary

Support for group therapy (other than CBT) for treating chronic pain patients with multiple pain problems must be regarded as tentative at best and poor at worst. There is not only a conspicuous absence of any RCTs, there is not much support for it empirically or qualitatively. Yet, all the proponents are emphatic in their support for incorporating group therapy, in one form or another, into the overall treatment plan for our patients. There is significant clinical support for that position, but this level of optimism must be supported by objective evidence. In the following sections we examine the efficacy of group therapy in relation to two specific pain disorders: fibromyalgia and headache.

Group Therapy and Fibromyalgia

In this group we present six reports of the efficacy of group therapy for fibromyalgia. All the studies had a comparison group and, in broad terms, reported a positive outcome. Kogstad and Hintringer (1993) compared 71 patients with confirmed diagnosis of fibromyalgia with 71 patients matched with the age, sex, and pain score based on a visual analogue scale. All patients were referred by family physicians. A number of valid instruments were used at assess outcome.

The classes had weekly 2-hour sessions and the topics were education, exercise/physical training, demonstration of relaxation techniques, and group discussion. Communication and problem solving were also incorporated into the group sessions. Family members were invited to attend one of the sessions. A specially trained physiotherapist conducted the classes.

The results were positive. At 1-year follow-up, subjects in the experimental group had significantly better global scores than the controls. Many of the scores on social and family matter, such as social withdrawal, satisfaction in general with life, family problems, easier contact with others, and level of relaxation, were better for the experimental group, but not statistically significant. The average use of healthcare services was reduced by 10% for the treatment group, which was not statistically significant. The number of subjects returning to work for the treatment group was from 5 to 15, and for the control group it fell from 23 to 12. However, it must be noted that on the SIP Scale the groups failed to attain statistically significant differences. The authors concluded that a "structured pain school" could serve as a supplement to other treatment modalities to treat patients with fibromyalgia and indeed other chronic pain sufferers. Nevertheless, more clinical trials were called for.

Burckhardt et al. (1994) investigated the effectiveness of education and physical therapy in the treatment of fibromyalgia. Ninety women with fibromyalgia were randomly assigned to one of three groups: (1) The education-only group received a 6-week self-management course; (2) the education plus physical training group received the educational program and 6 hours of physical training to help patients develop the ability to exercise independently; and (3) the control group received treatment after 3 months. In effect, this was a WLC. Eighty-seven patients completed the treatment.

Both experimental programs showed significant improvements in their quality of life and self-efficacy. At 6 weeks, the point of termination of the program, the patients showed a significant reduction in their report of helplessness, physical dysfunction, the number of days of feeling bad, and pain in the tender points. Long-term follow-up of 67 treated subjects revealed that 87% of the subjects were exercising at least three times a week for 20 minutes or more; 70% were practicing relaxation techniques, 46% were employed half-time as opposed to 37% at pretest. The authors concluded that self-efficacy of the treated subjects was enhanced significantly.

This investigation involved 32 patients with confirmed diagnosis of fibromyalgia (Keel et al., 1998). They were randomly assigned to either the experimental or the control group. Each group consisted of eight patients. The objectives of treatment in the experimental group were to enable the patients to gain mastery over their pain, to accept pain as something to live with, and to abandon the idea of a miracle cure. The experimental group program consisted of 15 weekly group sessions of 2 hours' duration and each session consisted of information, instruction in self-control strategies, gymnastics, relaxation, and group discussion. Control groups were instructed only in autogenic training. A wide range of valid instruments were used to measure outcome, and patients were also asked to maintain a diary. Of the 32 patients, 3 dropped out, 1 refused to participate in the active part of the program, 1 refused posttreatment tests, and 1 failed to complete the questionnaires due to poor skills in German. Finally, the number of patients completing the program stood at 27.

The outcome showed a number of improvements in the experimental group when compared with the control group, but not in the statistically significant range. For instance, at follow-up, the experimental group showed a reduction in medication consumption and in physical therapies, less sleep disturbance, and an improvement in the pain score, global assessment, and general symptoms, but differences lacked statistical significance. Only five patients attained measurable success at follow-up, and comparing these 5 with 22 cases revealed that their duration of pain was significantly less than the rest. None of them had a disability pension, suggesting they were more functional. They also showed more initiative for conflict resolution and were more active before the onset of treatment.

The authors concluded that only a small number of patients with lasting clinical improvement could be identified. Although psychological intervention combined with physiotherapy could be beneficial, it only seemed to apply to a selected group of a relatively small number of patients. Patients who had suffered from fibromyalgia for a longer time apparently had fallen too much into passivity and resignation, making it difficult for them to change.

Mueller and colleagues (2003) reported testing a German version of the Arthritis Self-Efficacy Short-Form Scale (ASES). This is not a strictly an outcome study, but validation of ASES. In the process, however, the efficacy of group therapy was indirectly established. The sample consisted of 43 female patients with fibromyalgia. Group treatment consisted of 12 weekly sessions, 90 minutes each over a 9-week period. Six patients dropped out and eight were excluded for missing data. Self-efficacy and expectations concerning pain and other disease-related symptoms were assessed with the eight-item short version of the ASES. In addition, locus of control, pain levels, general beliefs, functional capacity depression, and coping were measured using established and valid instruments.

This study established the suitability of using the ASES for measuring disease-related self-efficacy in fibromyalgia patients. Their conclusion was that the application of the ASES confirmed the hypothesis that self-efficacy could be enhanced by integrating psychological and physical group therapy in patients with fibromyalgia. Because validation of an instrument was in a different language, there was no report on follow-up.

The final study in this section compared the efficacy of group therapy with a WLC for patients with fibromyalgia, which had elements of CBT, anger management, and communication skills (Stillman, 2006). Forty-six patients were randomly assigned to a 4-week experimental group therapy and a WLC. The WLC received treatment upon completion of therapy for the experimental group.

The outcome data revealed that significant results were achieved in the following areas: mental health, communication, vitality, and pain management. The results confirmed the effectiveness of a short-term group intervention in treating specific issues that may confront patients with fibromyalgia.

Summary

The effectiveness of group therapy for fibromyalgia was generally confirmed by the studies discussed here. There was a major exception where the findings were less than encouraging (Keel et al., 1998). Only 5 of 22 patients benefited from group therapy. The question of patient selection remains an open issue, and very little evidence about patient characteristics that may predict positive outcome for group intervention with fibromyalgia patients emerged from this review. Yet, the data support the effectiveness of group therapy with this patient population.

Group Therapy for Headache Sufferers

We report three studies here. All of them had a control condition. Figueroa (1982) compared the effectiveness of (1) a behavioral package, which consisted of learning skills that enabled them to deal successfully with stressful and demanding situations, relaxation skills, and pain control techniques; (2) traditional psychotherapy; and (3) self-monitoring. Fifteen subjects with tension-type headache were randomly assigned to the three treatment conditions.

The behavior group received a three-stage program over seven 90-minute sessions. The psychotherapy group's treatment consisted of seven 90-minute sessions. The focus was to improve interpersonal relations that might have been contributing to conflicts. Participants were encouraged to discuss current stressful events. The self-monitoring group, in effect a WLC, was asked to maintain a self-monitoring form, same as that of the other two groups. They were told when their treatment would commence, and were encouraged to maintain an accurate record.

Results showed that virtually on all measures the behavior group showed a significant improvement over the other two groups. Frequency and duration of pain, degree of disability due to pain, medication taken, and relaxation were all significantly reduced when compared with the other two groups. There were no significant differences between the psychotherapy group and the self-monitoring group. However, it is noteworthy that all subjects in both treatment conditions reported a decrease in their headache activity despite the fact that the psychotherapy group experienced only nominal and nonsignificant change.

Finn et al. (1991) reported on the effectiveness of rational emotive therapy in treating muscle contraction headaches. Subjects included a community sample, and 35 respondents met the criteria for inclusion. There were 12 men and 23 women with the mean age of almost 33 years. The duration of pain ranged from 6 months to 40 years.

Following the screening, subjects were randomly assigned to four groups: (1) the rational emotive therapy (RET) group; (2) the progressive muscle relaxation (PMR) group; (3) the headache discussion (HAD) group; and (4) the WLC group. The outcome was measured in terms of weekly duration of headache, frequency, severity, and the number of headache-free days.

The treatment consisted of 10 weekly, $1^1/_2$-hour group sessions. All 35 subjects completed the program. The results revealed that headache duration approached significance, as did severity. RET and PMR were equally effective and produced better results than HAD and waiting list. At 2-month follow-up none of the outcome measures reached significance. The authors concluded that RET and PMR were useful strategies in reducing the frequency and severity of muscle contraction headache. They attributed the failure of headache-free days and headache duration to achieve statistical significance to methodological factors and the relatively small sample size. Nevertheless, the results of this study were equivocal.

McGrady and associates (1994) reported on the effectiveness of biofeedback-assisted relaxation (BR) in the treatment of migraine. The control group was required to relax by themselves, termed as "self-relax." The sample consisted of

23 patients with confirmed diagnosis of migraine. They were randomly assigned to one of the two groups. The experimental group consisted of 11 and the control group of 12 patients. Experimental patients received 12 sessions of biofeedback over a 12-week period. The self-relax group was to relax on their own for 10–15 minutes twice daily, concentrating on peaceful thoughts or on their breathing. The outcome was measured in terms of the reduction in the cerebral blood flow.

Main effects analysis showed that the experimental group had lower forehead muscle tension and increased finger temperature, whereas the control group failed to register such changes. In the experimental group pain reduced by 35%, whereas in the control group pain reduced by only 7.7%. On the psychological measures of anxiety and depression, decreases were observed in both groups but did not reach statistically significant values. The authors concluded that the results of this study confirmed that the biofeedback-assisted relaxation therapy was superior to self-relaxation in reducing pain and medication intake. A point of note is that the therapies employed in this study were more in the psychophysiological domain rather in the strictly psychosocial domain. Yet, as a brief group intervention, biofeedback-assisted relaxation was shown to have merit.

Summary

Two of the three studies reported positive outcome with behaviorally oriented group therapy. Rational emotive therapy in treating muscle contraction headache, while demonstrating some level of effectiveness, failed to be significantly different from control treatment conditions. The actual number of studies is far too small to make any definitive claims about the effectiveness of group therapy for headaches. Another omission, already noted, was the limited range of therapy (exclusively behavioral). One fact that may be worthy of note is that meta-analytic reviews of the literature have consistently shown that behavioral interventions yield 35–55% improvements, and these outcomes are significantly superior to control conditions (Rains et al., 2005).

Conclusion

One of the arguments for implementing group therapy is supposed to be its cost-effectiveness. If the same amount of time and person-power can be invested in treating a number of individuals rather than one patient at a time, then group therapy makes good economic sense. However, collective findings on the differential effectiveness of group therapy when compared with individual-based interventions remain problematic. McRoberts and colleagues (1998) conducted a meta-analysis of 23 outcome studies that directly compared the effectiveness of group and individual interventions when they were used within the same study. The results indicated no difference in the outcome between the two forms of interventions. Their findings bolster the cost-effective argument in favor of group therapy.

This chapter reviewed the effectiveness of group therapy (excluding CBT) for medical illness, depression, mixed pain condition, fibromyalgia, and headache. Overall, the actual number of research studies involving group therapy and chronic pain conditions is few as they are with medically ill patients. The results are not altogether encouraging. For example, group therapy was found to be effective only with uncomplicated depression. We also examined the effectiveness of social support intervention only to discover its lack of use with chronic pain populations. The results with mixed pain and headache were also far from encouraging.

On the contrary, there was reason for optimism for group therapy with fibromyalgia. Overall, the studies confirmed the effectiveness of group therapy over control conditions. One reason for the very limited use of group therapy methods other than CBT in treating chronic pain conditions can, in part, be explained by the very popularity of CBT. One major omission noted in the body of research reviewed here was the lack of information on patient characteristics that may predict positive outcome. Much work remains to be done in that respect.

References

Baines, L., Joseph, J., and Jindal, R. (2004) Prospective randomized study of individual and group psychotherapy versus group psychotherapy versus controls in recipients of renal transplants. Kidney Int., 65: 1937–1942.

Boyle, G. and Ciccone, V. (1994) Relaxation alone in combination with rational emotive therapy: effects on mood and pain. Pain Clin., 7: 253–265.

Burckhardt, C., Mannerkorpi, K., Hedenberg, L., and Bjelle, A. (1994) A randomized controlled trial of education and physical training for women with fibromyalgia. J. Rheumatol., 21: 714–720.

Cain, E., Kohorn, E., Quianlan, D., et al. (1986) Psychosocial benefits of a cancer support group. Cancer, 57: 183–189.

Dahl, J. and Fallstrom, C. (1989) Effects of behavioral group therapy on pain. Scand. J. Behav. Ther., 18: 137–143.

DeGoody, D. and de Godoy, R. (2003) A randomized controlled trial of the effect of psychotherapy on anxiety and depression in chronic obstructive pulmonary disease. Arch. Phys. Med. Rehabil., 84: 1154–1157.

Dolce, J., Crocker, M., and Doleys, D. (1986) Prediction of outcome among chronic pain patients. Behav. Res. Therapy, 24: 313–319.

Engels, G. and Vermy, M. (1997) Efficacy of non-medical treatments of depression in elders: a quantitative analysis. J. Geropsycol., 3: 17–35.

Figueroa, J. (1982) Group treatment of chronic tension headaches: a comparative treatment study. Behav. Modif., 6: 229–239.

Finn, T., DiGiuseppe, R., and Culver, C. (1991) The effectiveness of rational-emotive therapy in the reduction of muscle contraction headaches. J. Cogn. Psychother., 5: 93–103.

Gamsa, A., Braha, E., and Catchlove, R. (1985) The use of structured group therapy sessions in the treatment of chronic pain patients. Pain, 22: 91–96.

Hogan, B., Linden, W., and Najarian, B. (2002) Social support interventions: do they work? Clin. Psychol. Rev., 22: 381–440.

Keel, P., Bodoky, C., Gerhard, U., and Muller, W. (1998) Comparison of integrated group therapy and group relaxation training for fibromyalgia. Clin. J. Pain, 14: 232–238.

Kelly, J., Murphy, D., Bahr, G., et al. (1993) Outcome of cognitive behavioral and support group brief therapies for depressed HIV-positive patients. Am. J. Psychiatry, 150: 1679–1686.

Kleinke, C. (1987) Clients' preference for pain treatment modalities in a multidisciplinary pain clinic. Rehabil. Psychol., 32: 113–120.

Kogstad, O. and Hintringer, F. (1993) Patients with fibromyalgia in pain school. J. Musculoskeletal Pain, 3–4: 261–265.

Lanza, A. and Revenson, T. (1993) Social support interventions for rheumatoid arthritis: the cart before the horse? Health Educ. Q., 20: 97–117.

Markowitz, J., Spielman, L., Sullivan, M., and Fishman, B. (2000) An exploratory study of ethnicity and psychotherapy outcome among HIV-positive patients with depressive symptoms. J. Psychother. Pract. Res., 9: 226–231.

McDermut, W., Miller, I., and Brown, R. (2001) The efficacy of group-psychotherapy for depression: a meta-analysis and review of the empirical research. Clin. Psychol. Sci. Prac., 8: 98–116.

McGrady, A., Wauquier, A., McNeil, A., and Gerard, G. (1994) Effects of biofeedback assisted relaxation on migraine headache and changes in cerebral blood flow velocity in the middle cerebral artery. Headache, 34: 424–428.

McRoberts, C., Burlingame, G., and Hoag, M. (1998) Comparative efficacy of individual and group psychotherapy: a meta-analytic perspective. Group Dyn., 2: 101–117.

Mueller, A., Hartmann, M., Mueller, K., and Eich, W. (2003) Validation of the arthritis self-efficacy short-form scale in German fibromyalgia patients. Eur. J. Pain, 7: 163–171.

Rahe, R., Ward, H., and Hayes, V. (1979) Brief group therapy in myocardial infarction rehabilitation: three to four year follow-up of a controlled trial. Psychosom. Med., 41: 229–242.

Rains, J., Penzien, D., McCrory, D., and Gray, R. (2005) Behavioral headache treatment: history, review of the empirical literature, and methodological critique. Headache, 45(Suppl. 2): s92–s109.

Roy, R. (2001) Social Relations and Chronic Pain. New York, Kluwer/Plenum Publishers.

Roy, R. (2007) Social Dislocation and Chronic Pain Patient. In: Bond, M. (Ed.) Encyclopedia of Pain. Berlin/Heidelberg, Springer/Verlag.

Stillman, A. (2006) The effects of anger management and communication training and quality of life status in fibromyalgia patients. Dissertation Abstracts International. Section B: The Sciences and Engineering. 67(2-B0): 1177.

Uchino, B., Uno, D., and Holt-Lunstad, J. (1999) Social support, physiological processes, and health. Curr. Direction Psychol. Sci., 8: 145–148.

Vamos, M. (2006) Psychotherapy in the medically ill: a commentary. Aust. New Z J. Psychiatry, 40: 295–309.

Van Dam, H., van der Horst, F., Knoops, L., Ryckman, R., Crebolder, H., and van den Borne, B. (2005) Social support in diabetes: a systematic review of controlled intervention studies. Patient Educ. Couns., 59: 1–12.

Weir, R., Woodside, D., and Crook, J. (1988) Group therapy for chronic pain patients: a view of complexity. Pain Clin., 2: 109–120.

Chapter 10
Multidisciplinary Approach and Chronic Pain

In the preceding chapters we have discussed specific psychosocial interventions. This chapter is a departure in the sense that here we propose to examine the efficacy of multidisciplinary interventions in the treatment of chronic pain either in an inpatient or in an outpatient setting. Reports of program evaluation abound in the literature. It is for this reason that our presentation is somewhat selective and arbitrary. For the most part, we report more recent literature. The most comprehensive review of the literature on the outcome of pain management programs to date confirms the overall efficacy of these programs to reduce pain, improve psychosocial functioning, and increase the probability of patients returning to work, and also their cost-effectiveness (Gatchel and Okifuji, 2006).

Multidisciplinary treatment programs vary a great deal in terms of both the number of disciplines involved and the mode and length of therapy. Group intervention is common, but not exclusive. Psychological and medical components are commonly the underpinning of these programs. Beyond that, however, the use of physical therapy, occupational therapy, message therapy, social work, rehabilitation counselor, recreational therapist may vary very considerably from treatment program to treatment program (Chen, 2006).

Outcome measures are also varied. Some programs are designed to promote return to work, whereas others are more concerned with improving the day-to-day functioning of the patients. Chen (2006) noted that short-term benefits of multidisciplinary treatment programs often include pain reduction, improved flexibility, trunk strength, tolerance, self-perceived health status, pain-related disability, and mood.

William (1988) had observed that the outcome measures for the multidisciplinary treatment were varied, and drawn from physiological, psychological, sociocultural, and economic. Together, they formed the definition of a chronic pain database that could help classify syndromes, assess patient suitability, and evaluate outcomes. However, as was observed by Donovan and associates (1999), many therapies were effective with the subgroups of the chronic pain population, but no therapy was consistently effective. Furthermore, the more therapies included in the pain management programs, the more likely it was that a given individual would find an intervention that was helpful. They listed the following therapies generally used for treating chronic pain: acupuncture, biofeedback, blocks, education, exercise,

R. Roy, *Psychosocial Interventions for Chronic Pain*,
DOI: 10.1007/978-0-387-76296-8_10 © Springer Science+Business Media, LLC 2008

manipulation, antidepressants, adjuvants, and a variety of analgesic drugs. All or some of these therapies are usually present in a multidisciplinary treatment program.

This chapter has three parts. First, we consider program evaluation for general chronic populations commonly encountered in pain clinics. Second, we review the program evaluation literature for CLBP. Our reason for conducting a separate review for the latter is that back pain is ubiquitous in the general population, and they are usually very well represented in pain clinic populations. Third, we present a brief review of the literature on the comprehensive approach to treat pain in the elderly, a rather neglected group.

Mixed Chronic Pain and Program Evaluation

We examine the first part in three sections: (1) program evaluations in which return to work is a specific goal; (2) a more general outcome related to pain management and psychosocial well-being; and (3) a brief excursion into the program evaluation for the elderly chronic pain sufferers.

Return to Work

Many previous reviews have demonstrated the efficacy of multidisciplinary programs in returning chronic pain sufferers to work. In this segment we report four studies that had return to work as a specific outcome measure (Baker et al., 2005; Dolce et al., 1986; Jankus, 1995; Skouen et al., 2006).

Dolce and associates (1986) reported on a study that examined the role of self-efficacy experiences as predictors of outcome in a group of 63 chronic pain patients who were consecutively treated in a behaviorally oriented multidisciplinary pain-management program. The subjects had an assortment of pain sites including head and neck, back and leg, foot, and abdomen. Treatment consisted of a 4-week program and included psychology, physical therapy, social work, occupational therapy, nursing, and neurology. The measures included Minnesota Multiphasic Personality Inventory (MMPI), Beck Depression Inventory (BDI), the patient's pain ratings, and ratings of self-efficacy and concern.

The results showed a significant reduction in depression, on several scales of the MMPI, and a lessening of concern for exercise, medication, and work. As for return to work, 82% of the subjects were unemployed at the inception of treatment and this was reduced to 40% at follow-up. Poorer follow-up work status was related to higher pretreatment pain ratings and higher posttreatment scores on BDI and MMPI. In short, patients who failed to return to work did not benefit form the treatment to any significant level. The authors noted that although clinicians have little control over patients' pretreatment pain levels, they may be able to improve the percentage of patients who return to work by targeting behavioral changes that might improve patients' heightened anticipatory anxiety.

The following study demonstrated the long-term benefits of a multidisciplinary pain management program for a group of injured workers who developed chronic pain conditions (Jankus et al., 1995). This was a retrospective review of the long-term benefit of treatment for injured workers with chronic pain. A chart review was conducted for 233 patients who had sustained industrial injury. Of these, 158 patients were enrolled in a comprehensive outpatient interdisciplinary pain program. The treatment team comprised a physician, a physical therapist, an occupational therapist, and "psychosocial staff."

The authors were particularly interested in determining subjective pain improvement between the beginning and end of the treatment program, maintenance of pain improvement, usefulness of the program in managing their pain, and return to work. Questionnaires were mailed to 139 patients who had completed the program. In all, 91 patients responded and the analysis is based on these patients.

The results showed that 93% patients reported a reduction in their pain upon completion of the program. However, this had declined to 76% 3 years later in the survey. As for return to work, at initial evaluation 47 patients were not working; 35 reported returning to work or being involved in retraining. An important finding that emerged from the analysis was that significantly more patients are likely to return to work if referred early following the accident. In other words, delay in referral reduced the probability of returning to work. The authors concluded that based on their data, the interdisciplinary pain management program proved effective for the majority of patients in terms of both reducing pain and returning to work.

Our next report is a large-scale report of an RCT of 208 patients with chronic widespread pain (CWP) who, on average, were on sick leave for 3 months (Skouen et al., 2006). Patients were randomly allocated to the "extensive" program including group sessions, education, exercise training, and infrequent workplace intervention that lasted 4 weeks with a 6-hour session, 5 days a week; a light and individual program that consisted of an hour-long lecture on anatomy, pain mechanisms, exercise training, and life style; and a TAU group. The number of days of absence from work and full return to work were used as outcome measures, and the follow-up lasted for 54 months after the completion of treatment.

The results were revealing. In the first place, independent of the type of treatment, women and men with poor prognosis were absent from work more days compared with those with good prognosis. Older persons were more likely to be absent from work. The extensive program was associated with significantly fewer days of absence from work among women. Among men too the light program was associated with more days of absence from work. However, the treatment effect of the extensive program weakened significantly after 1–2 years following the termination of the program. No clear explanation for this phenomenon emerged. Neither was the relationship between higher age and lower probability of returning to work amenable to easy explanation. The main finding was that the extensive multidisciplinary program was more effective in returning women to work

Our final report is also an investigation into the effectiveness of a work-hardening program (Baker et al., 2005). This was a retrospective study based on chart reviews of patients referred to a Work Evaluation and Rehabilitation Clinic (WERC). This program was developed in 1994. Patients for inclusion in this program had to be medically stable, but unable to work in their preinjury job. A total of 196 patients whose records were found to be complete met the inclusion criteria. Of these 196 patients, 166 began the program, and 141 completed the WERC program.

The WERC program consisted of a 4-week, 6 hours per day treatment for 5 days a week in a work-like environment with the ultimate goal of returning the patients to their original job or employer. Treatment included medical, physiotherapy, occupational therapy, and discussion groups dealing with a multitude of issues ranging from anger management to family relationships and grief.

The results showed significant improvement on the five predictors of outcome, which included measures of daily living, grip strength, range of motion, pain and disability, and depression. A regression analysis revealed diagnosis, the level of education, gender and preinjury work history as significant predictors of outcome. The authors were careful to observe that regardless of the type of work-hardening program, the central goal must be reduction in pain and elevated functioning. The WERC program was shown to be effective posttreatment in all of the outcome measures.

Summary

All the studies had a number of common factors. They were, in the main, behaviorally oriented, and multidisciplinary components were more or less the same. The outcome was positive. The goal of these programs was singular in that the programs were specifically designed to return patients to work. All four studies reported some significant measure of success. The patient groups were, however, not homogeneous. They ranged from what may constitute a pain clinic population to injured workers to another group of workers absent from work with pain complaints. Nevertheless, it would appear that programs that are specifically designed for specific populations with the stated objective of returning them to work achieve a measurable level of success in attaining their goal. Gatchel and Okifuji (2006) estimated that the mean rate of return to work following comprehensive pain treatment was 66% compared with a mean rate of only 27% for conventional medical treatment. However, they also cautioned that return to work depended on a number of factors such as the age of the patient, the length of unemployment, economic environment, and regional variation.

Pain Management Programs and Psychosocial Well-Being

We report on four recent investigations that examined the efficacy of pain management programs in improving, in general terms, the quality of life for their patients (Chelminski et al., 2005; de Williams et al., 1996; Dysvik et al., 2004; Gupta et al., 2000).

Gupta and associates (2000) reported on the outcome of a residential pain management program (INPUT) involving 20 patients with chronic pain. Altogether, 25 patients were referred over a 2-year period. Of these, 20 completed treatment. Treatment consisted of CBT, physiotherapy, nursing, medicine, and occupational therapy. The residential program was delivered for 4 days a week for 4 weeks. The objectives were to improve fitness, return to more normal functioning, improve mood and stress management, and reduce negative effects of chronic pain on the family.

Upon completion of treatment, patients and their general practitioners (family physicians) were sent locally designed questionnaires; 18 patients and 16 general practitioners responded. Of the 18 patients, 17 reported improvements in their quality of life. All except one patient reported improvement in goal setting, pacing, exercise and stretching, and learning to manage their flare-ups. Of the 18 patients, only 3 were in part-time employment, 9 were not working, 4 were planning to work, and 2 were actively looking for work.

The general practitioners reported a reduced utilization of healthcare services and improvement in the quality of life of their patients. There was a high level of agreement between the general practitioners' assessment of the patient's improvement and patients' perceived improvement in quality of life. The authors noted that patients attending the program generally benefited and there were significant short-term to medium-term benefits.

This study employed a survey design. It did not have a comparison group. It was not clear from their report if they used standard instruments to assess outcome, or relied solely on patient and general practitioner feedback. The authors were cognizant of reporting biases. However, they argued that unlike other surveys, they had attempted to quantify the benefits. Despite some methodological issues, the INPUT program was successful in achieving many of its stated goals.

Dysvik and associates (2004) reported on the outcome study of an interdisciplinary outpatient program for a mixed group of chronic pain sufferers. A consecutive sample of 88 outpatients participated in this quasi-experimental investigation. They ranged in age between 27 and 66 years, with the average age being 47. Most of the patients were employed or on sick leave or in retraining programs. Only one-third of the subjects were on disability leave. The average duration of pain was 10 years. After initial assessment, 76 subjects fulfilled the criteria for inclusion in this project. Implementation of this study was preceded by a pilot project involving seven subjects to test the validity and feasibility of the treatment program and the appropriateness of the instruments selected for the study.

Intervention was offered in groups of 8–12 patients and they met for 3 hours per week for 8 weeks. The treatment team consisted of a psychologist, a physician, a physiotherapist, two nurses, and an occupational therapist. The main objectives of the intervention were for the patients to gain knowledge and skills to improve coping and the quality of life. A variety of outcome measures were used to measure changes in patients' physical and psychosocial functioning. Seventy-five patients completed the program.

Pretest and posttest scores were compared on coping, pain intensity, and health-related quality of life (HQRL). Significant improvements were noted in problem-focused and emotion-focused coping, reduction in pain, global mental health, vitality, social functioning, and physical functioning. Two-thirds of the patients reported significant satisfaction with the program. The therapeutic dialogue was the most successful component of the program and homework the least successful. The authors noted that the group approaches had some intrinsic benefits such as mutual support, feedback, and active participation. They also observed that their study was a replication of previous studies using similar interventions.

Chelminski and associates (2005) reported on a pain management program that was a departure from the usual multidisciplinary pain management programs. The treatment team consisted of internists, clinical pharmacists, and psychiatrists. The setting was an academic general medicine clinic. Eighty-five patients were enrolled in this program. Inclusion criteria included pain of 3 months' duration or more; also, the patients were required to be on opioid therapy or to consider this treatment. Attending and resident physicians were encouraged to refer patients with problems of pain control or misuse of opioids.

The baseline assessment included data on sociodemographics, medical history, the level of pain and disability, and depression. The central thrust of intervention was effective management of opioid medication and depression and other complex psychiatric conditions. Patients were required to sign a "medication contract."

At 3-month follow-up, pain levels had been reduced by 12–15%, which were statistically significant. There was also a significant reduction in depression. Twenty-seven patients seriously misused medication. Characteristics of patients who failed to complete the treatment included non-Caucasian origin, a history of drug abuse, worsening depression, and elevated pain scores at baseline. The authors noted the necessity of an RCT to determine whether these were real effects or represented a "secular" trend.

The following study in this section is also methodologically the most sound. This was an RCT study to test the efficacy of a multidisciplinary treatment program based on cognitive behavioral principles for chronic pain sufferers (de Williams et al., 1996). Subjects included 121 mixed chronic pain sufferers whose pain had significantly disrupted their lives and who were no longer responsive to conventional medical interventions. Patients were drawn from all over the United Kingdom.

Patients were randomly assigned by the throw of a dice to one of three treatment conditions: (1) 4-week inpatient pain management, $n = 43$; (2) 8 half-day per week outpatient pain management, $n = 45$; (3) and a WLC, $n = 33$. Goals of intervention were extensive and included improved fitness and flexibility, improvement in work, leisure, and social pursuits, pacing of activities, problem solving and control of unhelpful thoughts, drug reduction, relaxation, sleep management, and relapse prevention. Each of these categories included many subgoals.

Therapy was implemented by an anesthesiologist, a psychologist, a physiotherapist, a nurse, and an occupational therapist. Patients were assessed pretreatment, and 1 month after discharge, and treated patients were also assessed at 6 months and 1 year after discharge. We report the outcome in broad terms. Overall, both the inpatient and outpatient groups made changes in most variables than did the WLC group. The inpatient group, however, made greater gains than the outpatient group. Improvements in both the treatment groups were noted in relation to pain impact, depression, pain self-efficacy, catastrophizing, hopelessness, and several measures of physical performance. At 1-year follow-up the patterns of change were mostly the same, with highly significant improvements as compared to pretreatment on all measures except pain intensity, pain distress, and a physical measure of arm endurance. The authors concluded that the methodology used in this study clearly constituted a significant advance of the cognitive behavioral management of chronic pain.

Summary

The four studies reviewed above employed a rather diverse methodology, ranging from a survey design to an RCT. Both inpatient and outpatient settings were used. The population investigated in one study was somewhat of a departure from the usual chronic pain population generally seen in pain clinics (Chelminski et al., 2005). Their population was drawn from a general medicine clinic. De Williams and associates' (1996) study employed the most sophisticated design (RCT), and for that reason its findings must carry more weight. However, regardless of methodology, all four studies demonstrated the value of pain management programs in significantly improving the quality of life for most patients suffering from a multitude of pain complaints of a chronic nature. However, it is noteworthy that the overall benefits of comprehensive pain management programs have been repeatedly confirmed in many reviews and meta-analytic reports (Gatchel and Okifuji, 2006).

A rather diverse set of outcome measures were used to assess the outcome, although the goals of treatment were more or less the same, namely, reduction in pain and improved quality of life. In this context it is worthy of note that a meta-analysis of 109 studies conducted in 1989 concluded that mood and subjective symptoms consistently showed greater improvement than did pain intensity, pain duration, or frequency of pain (Malone and Strube, 1989). Interventions had a more profound impact on reducing fear and depression associated with pain, but pain relief remained elusive. That picture seems to have changed over time as pain reduction is often a stated goal of therapy, and as is evident in the reports discussed above, not beyond achievement. A meta-analysis of 65 studies only a few years later was able to demonstrate on average pain reduction of some 29% following comprehensive pain treatment (Flor et al., 1992).

There was further confirmation that comprehensive pain treatment had the capacity of reducing pain from 14–60% to an average of 20–30% (Gatchel and Okifuji, 2006). These figures were comparable to treatment with opioid for chronic pain, which produced on average a 30% reduction in pain. They also concluded that comprehensive pain programs were therapeutically efficacious and cost-effective. Data on the major outcome variables of self-reported pain, function, healthcare utilization and cost, medication use, work factors, and insurance claims were available, and the review categorically established that comprehensive pain programs offered the most efficacious and cost-effective, evidence-based treatment for chronic pain sufferers. A point worthy of note is that many countries outside of the United States, such as Denmark (Becker et al., 2000; Thomsen et al., 2002), France (Nizard et al., 2003), and Japan (Kitahara et al., 2006), have reported the effectiveness of comprehensive pain treatment programs. These programs had the same or similar multidisciplinary components, with an emphasis on restoration of function and improvement management of pain comparable with those in the United States. The effectiveness of comprehensive pain management programs seems to transcend language and cultural barriers.

Peat et al. (2001) conducted a rather unique survey of all chronic pain programs in the United Kingdom to determine their practice for follow-up of treated patients. Of 70 such programs 66 (94%) responded. Fifty-eight programs were finally selected for this project. In broad terms, the programs had a commitment to follow up outcome evaluations, but the variability among them was very substantial in terms of the length of follow-up, attendance rates, and outcome measurements. This raised significant questions about the ability of these programs to accurately determine the longer-term outcome of chronic pain sufferers. Forty-one of the 58 programs met the minimum criteria for program content (provision of physical reconditioning, posture and body mechanisms training, relaxation techniques, information and education about pain management, medication review, psychological interventions, return to activity in daily living). As for follow-up, on average, 60–80% of patients were accounted for at follow-up. The most common final follow-up points were 6 or 12 months, the range being 1 month to 3 years. The authors concluded that these findings raised questions about the consistency of follow-up evaluation across the United Kingdom and the current arrangements in some of the programs to know the long-term efficacy of the programs. This study is of particular importance if some level of uniformity is to be incorporated in both the scope of the range of interventions in comprehensive pain management programs and their long-term efficacy. A gap in our collective knowledge of the long-term outcome of comprehensive pain interventions continues to exist.

Pain Management Programs and the Elderly

It needs to be stated at the outset that a programmatic approach to treat chronic pain in the elderly is a much underreported topic in the literature. Literature search on this topic reveals a paucity of research, and an acknowledgment of that reality. In fact, this is an old problem spanning several decades and the inevitable conclusion that can be drawn is that a comprehensive approach to chronic pain management in the elderly is not an area of priority for researchers. Helm and associates (1996) noted that given the high rate of prevalence of chronic pain in this population, it was inexplicable that they rarely received attention from physicians and specialists in pain management. They described a multidisciplinary program designed to treat elderly chronic pain sufferers, and reported on their success in reducing pain, increasing activity, and improving mood in their patients.

Gibson and associates (1996) in their comprehensive review of the literature on pain management for the elderly echoed Helm's concern. They also observed that elderly patients were conspicuously absent from mainstream pain clinics. Unfortunately, this fact remains unaltered even today. In their review Gibson and associates

(1996) reported on 14 studies on treatment outcome for chronic pain in the elderly. Results reported by these studies were usually positive, and reduction in pain levels, increased activity, and lowering of depression were noted. These studies were all presentations at conferences, and information was derived from conference abstracts. Gibson and associates concluded their article on an optimistic note. Interest in pain issues in the elderly was on the rise, and the need for a multidisciplinary pain clinic for treating chronic pain in the elderly was starting to be recognized.

We identified a number of community-based programs to treat pain in geriatric patients that are worthy of attention (Austrian et al., 2005; Barry et al., 2004; Ersek et al., 2003; Kung et al., 2000; Lansbury, 2000). Barry and associates (2004) investigated the strategies used by the elderly to cope with chronic pain. Patients were recruited from a primary care practice located at a veterans hospital. A total of 245 patients participated in this study. A combination of qualitative and quantitative methods was used. Altogether, 240 patients had employed one or more strategies during the previous month. These strategies included analgesic medication used by 78% (187/240), exercise by 35%, cognitive methods by 37%, religious activities by 21%, and activity restriction by 20%. Pain medication was used mostly by patients with problems of joint and muscle pain. Exercise, on the contrary, was widely used except for trauma-related pain. The results showed that the perceived effectiveness of the coping strategies was modest, and efforts to maximize the benefits were called for.

The next study was almost an extension of the previous. This investigation probed into the barriers to self-management approaches for chronic pain in the geriatric population (Austrian et al., 2005). Subjects were recruited from an ambulatory geriatric treatment program and involved 68 participants. A qualitative method was employed to ascertain the barriers these patients encountered to participation. Only 16% of the patients reported engaging in exercise programs to manage pain, whereas a full 73% reported a willingness to do so. Relaxation was used by only 4%, but 70% reported a willingness to learn this technique. Investigators identified 17 barriers, which included time conflicts, transportation, treatment efficacy concerns, and fear of pain and injury. The authors urged addressing the removal of the barriers that would substantially increase the number of patients willing to take charge of their own pain management. These two community-based programs are important for the reason that community-dwelling elderly patients with chronic pain, in the first place, are willing to self-manage their chronic pain, and, second, removal of the barriers could only increase their level of participation.

Lansbury (2000) conducted a study that was in a similar vein as the two preceding reports. The point of this investigation was to ascertain the use of coping strategies and the barriers encountered. This was a qualitative study. Seventy-two participants were recruited using a purposive sampling technique and selected from six suburbs in Sydney, Australia. Samples were divided into young-old (65–70 years) and old-old (75 years and over). The criteria for inclusion were as follows: a subject aged 65 and over, living at home and speaking English. They also had to have a history of pain for 3 months or more. Data were collected in six focus groups, which ranged in size from 6 to 30. All recorded interviews were transcribed and analyzed using the constant comparative method in which the data were immediately analyzed and coded.

A vast majority of patients had musculoskeletal pain, the next group being patients with cardiovascular problems such as angina and stroke. Just above 24% of the subjects reported severe pain and nearly 41% mild pain. Preferred coping strategies were those that could be self-administered such as home remedies, massage and topical agents, physical agents, and informal cognitive strategies. The least favored were prescribed treatment, medications, physiotherapy, and exercise.

As for the barriers, cost ranked high, as did access to health care, side effects of medication, lack of information, the elderly person's attitude to pain, the attitude of the professional, fear of loss of control and independence, past negative experience, a dislike of diagnostic tests, and acceptance of their own pain. Lansbury (2000) concluded that older people could help manage their own pain if they had the opportunity to learn to be more assertive in asking for help. Beyond that there was a clear need for improvement in health services to meet the needs of older adults with chronic pain.

Another program that reported a community-based treatment program for elderly chronic pain sufferers involved 71 participants who received treatment and who were compared with an untreated group of 40 persons (Kung et al., 2000). A quasi-experimental design was used for this study. The treatment program was designed to help older people with chronic pain in acquiring a good understanding of their pain, its negative effects, and management options, and to improve access to services considered useful.

Participants were allowed to opt for more than one program. The community-based intervention had two elements. The first stage involved an educational seminar consisting of four sessions of 1-hour presentations that covered pain-related topics ranging from pain perception to medical and psychological approaches to manage pain. At the end of the educational programs, participants could choose from a wide range of interventions that included attending a pain management center, receiving help from allied health professionals, taking part in an exercise, relaxation or massage program, a self-management course and the use of transcutaneous nerve stimulation. Very wide-ranging outcome measures were employed to measure physical and psychosocial parameters.

The results showed that, on the whole, persons who participated in the programs showed significant improvements compared with those who did not. The educational program and the intervention choice resulted in a significant reduction in pain intensity and an increased physical activity for the participants. The results of a 6-month follow-up, however, revealed that only the benefits of physical activity were maintained. The treatment benefits were of a short-term nature. The authors recommended an RCT to fully understand the role of choice in the management of chronic pain and the implications for improving the effectiveness of the interventions.

The final report in this section also compared the efficacy of self-management of chronic pain in the elderly with that in a control group (Ersek et al., 2003). The subjects were independent living residents of three retirement communities. Inclusion criteria were as follows: (1) resident in one of the three communities;

(2) 60 years and older; (3) pain duration of 3 months or more; (4) ability to complete questionnaires (literate); and (5) ability to attend at least five sessions.

The sample consisted of 45 subjects, of whom 39 were women, with the mean age of 81.9 years. The most common pain conditions were osteoarthritis, old fractures, and neuralgia. A wide range of outcome measures were used to assess physical function, depression, and pain interference with activity. Another set of assessments were related to the process outcome. Participants completed all the instruments related to outcome at baseline, 9 weeks later, and 3 months after the posttreatment assessment. Subjects were randomly assigned to 7–90 minute group sessions conducted at the retirement facilities and given an educational booklet. The booklet was designed to assist participants in managing their pain more effectively, but it proved to be less effective than in the case of the self-management group.

The results were mixed. The self-management group showed significant improvement posttreatment in physical role function and pain intensity. However, on measures of pain-related activity interference, depression, and pain-related beliefs, the findings were nonsignificant. The authors concluded that the study provided preliminary support for a self-management group intervention program for older adults with chronic pain.

Summary

All the studies shared many common features. There was a clear recognition that the elderly pain sufferers encountered in pain clinics represented a subgroup of chronic pain sufferers. The need for more individualized interventions was clearly acknowledged. Most of the patients (as far as reported) suffered from musculoskeletal disorders, and a wide variety of noncancer pain. The range of interventions offered in these studies was varied, but the goals were similar. Control over pain and improved functioning were the two dominant objectives. Barriers to treatment were recognized, as was the need to make therapy accessible. One common conclusion was that the outcome, although favorable, had ample scope for improvement. One unstated conclusion to be derived from these reports is that the need for effective intervention with community-dwelling elderly pain sufferers remains largely unmet.

Multidisciplinary Approaches and CLBP

CLBP is perhaps the most ubiquitous among the chronic pain disorders. This condition is also more commonly presented in pain clinic settings. CLBP is recognized as one of the challenging problems that sometimes remains impervious to interventions. Yet, some of the more recent reviews and papers are beginning to present a more favorable outcome for comprehensive approaches to management of this critical pain condition.

Carragee (2005) noted that CLBP without sciatica, stenosis, or severe spinal deformity has a reported prevalence of 33%. In his search for various pharmacological and physical strategies to manage this pain in a particular patient with a history of back pain of 4 months' duration, he recognized that there was virtually no consensus on how to manage this very persistent problem. He provided a summary of pharmacological and nonpharmacological therapies, and injections and neuroablation procedures and surgery. His conclusion was that none of the methods of rehabilitation had consistently shown to have generalized applicability, and the long-term benefits remained unknown. Combination of medical care and physical therapy or manipulation could be moderately effective in reducing pain disability than any single therapy. In terms of treatment for his patient, he recommended a combination of an aggressive 3 to 6 weeks' rehabilitation program with functional and behavioral goals in combination with tricyclic antidepressants.

The last observation was a further confirmation of a review of the psychological literature for the treatment of CLBP (Bailey, 2002). This meta-analysis of 146 psychological interventions included a wide variety of approaches to back pain treatment. Overall, the effectiveness of psychological interventions was limited. As for any single mode of intervention, no treatment of choice emerged. Adding physical therapy and medical components, however, improved effectiveness. Patients on compensation did not do as well as the noncompensated patients. This point was also noted by Gatchel and Okifuji (2006).

The most recent meta-analysis of psychological interventions for CLBP arrived at the following critical conclusions: (1) cognitive behavioral and self-regulatory treatments were efficacious on their own; (2) multidisciplinary programs that had a psychological treatment component, compared with controls, were also found to have positive short-term effects on pain interference, and positive long-term effects on return to work; and (3) and multidisciplinary programs produced significantly better outcomes than unimodal treatments in behavioral outcomes and return to work, thus confirming earlier findings (Hoffman et al., 2007). The meta-analysis was based on 22 studies, published across 25 articles.

The following review on the efficacy of intervention for back pain was of a different order (Schonstein et al., 2003). It examined the literature on work-hardening programs for workers with back and neck pain. Eighteen RCTs were identified and 243 relevant contrasts were also reviewed. They found evidence for the effectiveness of these programs if they had a cognitive behavioral component. Combined therapies reduced the number of sick days lost at 12-month follow-up by an average of 45 days when compared with "usual care" by general practitioners for workers with chronic back pain. The authors unequivocally declared that for work-related outcomes there was little or no evidence for the effectiveness of any specific exercises that were not used in conjunction with CBT in reducing days lost due to acute or chronic back pain. These three reviews shared a critical conclusion in common. No single therapy, be it psychological, physical, or pharmacological, was sufficient to yield positive outcome in the treatment of CLBP.

Gatchel and Okifuji (2006) in their review found support for the effectiveness of comprehensive pain treatment programs for CLBP in providing long-term benefits. They cited two RCTs. One of these studies involved a 2-year follow-up and the other a 5-year follow-up (Fairbank et al., 2005; Friedrich et al., 2005). They also found evidence for the higher cost-effectiveness of comprehensive pain treatment programs when compared with surgery for back pain (Rasmussen et al., 2005; Rivero-Arias et al., 2005).

Finally, we present a few studies that provide further support for long-term effectiveness and cost-effectiveness of pain management programs as well as a few reports of innovative multidisciplinary treatment programs for CLBP that have proven successful.

Kaapa and associates (2006) evaluated the effectiveness of a "semi-intensive" multidisciplinary rehabilitation for patients with low-back pain in an outpatient setting. A total of 120 women working in a healthcare or social care setting with a history of nonspecific CLBP were randomly assigned to an experimental group program ($n = 59$) that comprised physical training, workplace interventions, back school, relaxation training, and CBT for stress management and a control group ($n = 61$) assigned to a physiotherapy that included exercise and passive treatment methods. The outcome measures included intensity of pain, disability, sick leave, healthcare utilization, depressive symptoms, and beliefs of working ability after 2 years.

The results revealed virtually no significant differences between the two groups at 6, 12, and 24 months follow-up. Surprisingly, both groups maintained their improvements at 2-year follow-up. The authors concluded that a physiotherapy intervention with some cognitive orientation was just as effective as a multidisciplinary approach in maintaining the favorable effects over time. It should be noted that patients in this program were far more functional (employed) unlike many of the CLBP patients encountered in pain clinics. Nevertheless, the fact that a less costly intervention was able to achieve the same level of improvement over time does offer an alternative for patients who may not be seriously disabled by their back pain. This study successfully demonstrated both cost-effectiveness and relatively long-term outcome in the treatment of a subgroup of CLBP sufferers.

Another study arrived at a conclusion similar to that of the preceding report. A cost–utility analysis of physiotherapy treatment was compared with physiotherapy advice for CLBP (Rivero-Arias et al., 2006). The sample consisted of 286 patients with current persistent low-back pain who were randomly assigned to the two treatment conditions. Cost-effectiveness was expressed as the incremental cost per quality-adjusted life year gained. The total cost was not significantly different for the two groups. However, patients in the physiotherapy group had significantly higher out-of-pocket healthcare expenditure. Utility levels improved in both groups from a baseline to 12 months, with no significant difference between them. Given the higher out-of-pocket expenses for the physiotherapy group, advice given by a physiotherapist should be the first option.

The next study is unique in that it incorporated a plan for a truly long-term (13-year) follow-up in assessing the success of a multidisciplinary approach to treat CLBP (Patrick et al., 2004). Forty-five subjects, with CLBP and unable to work between 3 and 30 months, for this study originally participated in an RCT (Altmaier et al., 1992). These subjects were randomly assigned either to a standard 3-week inpatient treatment that had a large multidisciplinary component or to a psychological treatment, in which standard treatment in addition to a wide variety of CBTs for pain management was administered. In the current study an effort was made to contact all 45 patients 13 years after the termination of treatment. Of the 45 patients 28 were located and 26 agreed to participate in a telephone interview.

Patients were assessed on a wide array of outcome measures. Thirteen patients were working at the point of follow-up. Negative mood, which had increased from pretreatment to posttreatment, had, in fact, decreased over this long period of time. There was not a significant decrease in the domain of pain interference posttreatment and long-term follow-up. However, patients reported a significant lowering of their pain level between posttreatment and long-term follow-up. The study sample reported significantly greater pain than the general population and contrary to prediction these patients scored significantly more on physical functioning and role-physical.

The authors concluded that at least those patients who participated in the follow-up were able to maintain their short-term gains over a very long period. This was achieved despite the fact that the patients had grown considerably older. Another point of note was that most of these patients did not participate in additional treatment following the multidisciplinary intervention. Overall, the data lent support to the long-term effectiveness of multidisciplinary pain programs for the treatment of a subgroup of CLBP patients.

Van der Roer and associates (2004) evaluated the cost-effectiveness of an intensive group training program vis-à-vis physiotherapy for a group of subacute and CLBP patients. In an RCT the cost-effectiveness of the two modes of intervention would be evaluated. Simultaneously, a full economic evaluation would be conducted. The outcome of this study would be one of the very first to systematically address the question of cost-effectiveness. The authors noted that the no trials were available on cost-effectiveness and cost-utility.

Unusual Programs

We provide two examples of innovative approaches to therapy. A German study compared the effectiveness of a multidisciplinary rehabilitation program (MRP) and usual care for CLBP patients (Lang et al., 2003). Patients were recruited from independent physicians in the community who agreed to participate in this study. MRP involved 4 hours per day, 3 days a week for 20 days, and included restorative exercise therapy, physiotherapy, CBT, progressive muscle relaxation, and education. A wide range of outcome measures were used. One hundred and fifty-seven patients participated in the usual care program and 51 in the MRP group.

The MRP group showed significant improvement in physical and mental health measures as compared with the TAU patients. Days off work was also significantly lowered in the MRP group. On measures of overall appraisal of outcome, the MRP group scored significantly higher than the controls. However, no significant differences on measures of depression and pain-related interference emerged between the two groups. The authors, while advocating the MRP as a way of treating CLBP, cautioned that the MRP should be subjected to RCTs before wider application. The uniqueness of this program lay in the fact that care was provided by local healthcare providers in the community. Authors opted for this approach as multidisciplinary pain clinics are not available in every community, and they are limited by the number of patients they can treat. They provided a blueprint for a comprehensive approach to pain management utilizing community resources.

The next report examined the effectiveness of an interdisciplinary back educa- tion and evaluation program in improving patient's health-related quality of life (Claiborne et al., 2002). A total of 153 subjects participated in this study. All pa- tients had lumbar spine disease diagnosis caused by disease or injury. Patients were selected for either the back education and education program (n = 92) or the clinic program (n = 61). The back education program was a 4-day outpatient-based in- terdisciplinary education regime designed to empower patients through a process of assessment, education, and skill development, all resulting in a better quality of life. This was not a controlled study.

The two groups were different in many respects, one significant aspect being the higher level of disease and disability in the back education group when com- pared with a better functioning group in the clinic program. The results showed that the back education program patients improved in their physical quality of life. There was no improvement in the comparison group. Factors such as diminished disability, male gender, surgery during treatment, not receiving worker's compensa- tion, and susceptibility to depression predicted a favorable outcome. However, back treatment had no measurable effect on the mental component of the program. The striking aspect of this program, despite obvious methodological shortcomings, was the brevity of the program. It was delivered, albeit on an intensive basis, over a very short period of time. Unfortunately, there does not appear to be any replication of this approach utilizing an RCT design to fully explicate its value.

Summary

First and foremost, the effectiveness of a multidisciplinary approach to the treatment of CLBP has considerable validity. Review after review, more or less, demonstrate that the multidisciplinary approach is invariably superior to any other intervention, be it physical or psychosocial. Long-term benefits, although confirmed by a number of studies, are hard to locate on follow-up beyond 24 months. There was one study that reported the benefits of treatment being sustained after 13 years. A replication of this study may be instructive.

The costs and benefits of a multidisciplinary approach to CLBP are not always self-evident. Often, the evidence is indirect, but it still remains, by and large, an underresearched area. However, the fact is that the multidisciplinary approach has been shown to be superior over any other therapy and there truly is no alternative.

Finally, we presented two examples of innovative approaches: one involved a community endeavor to provide multidisciplinary treatment for CLBP in the ab- sence of an organized pain clinic and the other was impressive for the brevity of therapy, which led to significant improvements.

Conclusion

This chapter provides a broad overview on the effectiveness of multidisciplinary approaches to treating chronic pain. A telling conclusion that can be drawn from the body of research discussed above is that there does not appear to be any alternative to this comprehensive approach if any meaningful and significant improvement in our patients' lives is to be achieved. We examined its effectiveness in enabling patients to return to work and improve their quality of life and in treating elderly and CLBP sufferers. In each of these categories, the effectiveness of a comprehensive approach proved superior to any control conditions.

One area that requires further exploration is the long-term effectiveness of multidisciplinary treatment. We found one study that managed, albeit with some limitations, to conduct a follow-up 13 years after the termination of treatment. The results were encouraging. Another issue that confronts many communities in Canada and the United States is the question of access to these programs. They tend to exist in major centers often connected with medical schools. Waiting lists for admission can be formidable. In my own clinic, patients, on average, wait 2 years from the time of referral. We reported on one innovative community-based program that found an ingenious way of providing comprehensive care to chronic pain patients by coordinating community resources. That or some version of that could serve as a blueprint for further development of such programs.

References

Altmaier, M., Lehmann, T., and Russell, D. (1992) The effectiveness of psychological interventions for the rehabilitation of low back pain. Pain, 49: 377–387.

Austrian, J., Kerns, R., and Reid, M. (2005) Perceived barriers to trying self-management approaches for chronic pain in older persons. J. Am. Geriatr. Soc., 53: 856–861.

Bailey, G. (2002) The psychological treatment of back-pain: a meta-analysis. Dissertation Abstracts International. Section B. The Sciences and Engineering, 63(1-B): 515.

Baker, P., Goodman, G., Ekelman, B., and Bonder, B. (2005) The effectiveness of a hardening program as measured by lifting capacity, pain scales, and depression scores. Work, 24: 21–31.

Barry, L., Kerns, R., Guo, D., et al. (2004) Identification of strategies used to cope with chronic pain in older persons receiving primary care from a Veterans Medical Center. J. Am. Geriatr. Soc., 52: 950–956.

Becker, N., Sjojgren, P., Bech, P., et al. (2000) Treatment outcome of chronic non-malignant pain patients managed in a Danish multidisciplinary pain center compared to general practice: a randomized controlled trial. Pain, 84: 203–211.

Carragee, E. (2005) Persistent low-back pain. N. Engl. J. Med., 18: 1891–1898.

Chelminski, P., Ives, T., Felix, K., et al. (2005) A primary-care, multidisciplinary disease management program for opioid-treated patients with chronic non-cancer pain and a high burden of psychiatric co-morbidity. BMC Health Serv. Res., 5: 1–13.

Chen, J. (2006) Out-patient pain rehabilitation programs. Iowa Orthop. J., 26: 102–106.

Claiborne, N., Vandenburgh, H., Krause, T., and Leung, P. (2002) Measuring quality of life changes in individuals with chronic low back pain conditions: a back education program evaluation. Eval. Program Plann., 25: 61–70.

de Williams, A., Richardson, P., Nicholas, M., et al. (1996) Inpatient vs. outpatient pain management: results of a randomized controlled trial. Pain, 66: 13–22.

Dolce, J., Crocker, M., and Doleys, D. (1986) Prediction of outcome among chronic pain patients. Behav. Res. Ther., 3: 313–319.

Donovan, M., Evers, K., Jacobs, P., and Mandleblatt, S. (1999) When there is no benchmark: designing a primary care chronic pain management program from the scientific basis up. J. Pain Symptom Manage., 18: 38–48.

Dysvik, E., Vinsnes, A., and Eikeland, O. (2004) The effectiveness of a multidisciplinary pain management programme managing chronic pain. Int. J. Nurs. Pract., 10: 224–234.

Ersek, M., Turner, J., McCurry, S., et al. (2003) Efficacy of a self-management group intervention for elderly persons with chronic pain. Clin. J. Pain, 19: 156–167.

Fairbank, J., Frost, H., Wilson-MacDonald, J., et al. (2005) Randomized controlled trial to compare surgical stabilization of the lumbar spine with an intensive rehabilitation program for patients with chronic low-back pain. Br. Med. J., 330: 1233.

Flor, H., Fydrich, T., and Turk, D. (1992) Efficacy of multidisciplinary pain treatment centers: a meta-analytic review. Pain, 49: 221–230.

Friedrich, M., Gittler, G., Arendasy, M., and Friedrich, K. (2005) Long-term effect of a combined exercise and motivational program on the level of disability of patients with chronic low-back pain. Spine, 30: 995–1000.

Gatchel, R. and Okifuji, A. (2006) Evidence-based scientific data documenting the treatment and cost-effectiveness of comprehensive pain programs for nonmalignant pain. J. Pain, 7: 779–793.

Gibson, S., Farrell, M., Katz, B., and Helme, R. (1996) Multidisciplinary management of chronic nonmalignant pain in older adults. In: B. Ferrell and B Ferrell (Eds.) Pain in the Elderly (pp. 91-100). Seattle, IASP Press.

Gupta, S., Francis, J., Porter, G., and Valentine, J. (2000) An independent assessment of a supra regional pain management program and comparison of patients' and general practitioners' perceptions of their effect. Anesthesia, 55: 374–384.

Helm, R., Katz, B., Bradbeer, M., et al. (1996) Multidisciplinary pain clinic for old people: do they have a role? Clin. Geriatr. Med., 12: 563–582.

Hoffman, B., Papas, R., Chatkoff, D., and Kerns, R. (2007) Meta-analysis of psychological interventions for chronic low-back pain. Health Psychol., 26: 1–9.

Jankus, W., Park, T., VanKeulen, M., and Weisensel, M. (1995) Interdisciplinary treatment of the injured worker with chronic pain: long term efficacy. Wis. Med. J., 94: 244–249.

Kaapa, E., Frantsi, K., Sarna, S., and Malmivaara, A. (2006) Multidisciplinary group rehabilitation versus individual physiotherapy for chronic non-specific low back pain. Spine, 15: 371–376.

Kitahara, M., Kojima, K., and Ohmura, A. (2006) Efficacy of interdisciplinary treatment for chronic nonmalignant pain patients in Japan. Clin. J. Pain, 22: 647–655.

Kung, F., Gibson, S., and Helm, R. (2000) A community-based program that provides free choice of intervention for older people with chronic pain. Pain J., 1: 293–308.

Lang, E., Liebig, K., Kastner, S., et al. (2003) Multidisciplinary rehabilitation versus usual care for chronic low-back pain in the community: effects on quality of life. Spine, 3: 270–276.

Lansbury, G. (2000) Chronic pain management: a qualitative study of elderly people's preferred coping strategies and barriers to management. Disabil. Rehabil., 22: 2–14.

Malone, M. and Strube, M. (1989) Meta-analysis of non-medical treatments for chronic pain, Pain, 34: 231–244.

Nizard, J., Lombrail, P., Potel, G., et al. (2003) Evaluation of l'efficacite of the taken charge of 46 chronic pain by a treatment center of the pain. Douleur et Analgesie, 16: 187–196.

Patrick, L., Altmaier, E., and Found, E. (2004) Long-term outcomes in multidisciplinary treatment of chronic low back pain: results of a 13 year follow-up. Spine, 15: 850–855.

Peat, G., Moores, L., Goldingay, S., and Hunter, M. (2001) Pain management program follow-ups. A national survey of current practice in the United Kingdom. J Pain Symptom Manage., 21: 218–226.

Rasmussen, C., Nielsen, G., Hansen, V., et al. (2005) Disc surgery before and after implementation of multidisciplinary non-surgical spine clinic. Spine, 30: 2469–2473.

Rivero-Arias, O., Campbell, H., Gray, A., et al. (2005) Surgical stabilization of the spine compared with a program of intensive rehabilitation for the management of patients with chronic low-back pain: cost utility analysis based on a randomized controlled trial. Br. J. Med., 330: 1239.

Rivero-Arias, O., Gray, A., Frost, H., et al. (2006) Cost-utility analysis of routine physiotherapy treatment compared with physiotherapy advice in low back pain. Spine, 31: 1381–1387.

Schonstein, E., Kenny, D., Keating, J., and Koes, B. (2003) Work conditioning, work hardening and functional restoration for workers with back and neck pain. Cochrane Database Syst. Rev., 3.

Skouen, J., Grasdal, A., and Haldersen, M. (2006) Return to work after comparing outpatient multidisciplinary treatment programs versus treatment in general practice with chronic widespread pain. Eur. J. Pain, 10: 145–152.

Thomsen, A., Sorensen, J., Sjogrenm P., and Eriksen, J. (2002) Chronic non-malignant pain patients and economic consequences. Eur. J. Pain, 6: 342–352.

Van der Roer, N., van Tulder, M., Barendse, J., et al. (2004) Cost-effectiveness of an intensive group therapy training protocol compared to physiotherapy guideline care for sub-acute and chronic low back pain; design of a randomized controlled trial. BMC Musculoskelet. Disord., 5: 45–52.

William, R. (1988) Towards a set of reliable and valid measures for chronic pain assessment and treatment. Pain, 35: 239–251.

Chapter 11
Epilogue

All our comments and observations discussed in this chapter are directly related to medical illness in general and chronic pain in particular. We had two major objectives in writing this book. The first was to get a general idea of the types of psychotherapy in use to treat medically ill patients in general and pain patients in particular. We also considered the literature on depression and psychotherapy because it is commonly seen in chronic pain sufferers. The second was to ascertain the extent to which the practice of psychotherapy with medically ill persons in general and chronic pain sufferers in particular was evidence driven. On the first issue, although books and articles abound on the value of psychotherapeutic intervention with the medically ill, that cannot be said for chronic pain (Fisher and O'Donohue, 2006; McDaniel et al., 1992). For this reason, we decided to broaden our base and made a case that, by extrapolation, such therapies could be used for patients with chronic pain. An example of that would be our decision to include interpersonal psychotherapy (IPT). As for our second objective, we were somewhat disappointed. The scientist-practitioner model of practice for psychotherapy remains a challenge.

On the contrary, the justifiable popularity of CBT appears to be almost entirely rooted in the empirical support provided by RCTs. Although we have argued that CBT is not a panacea, which it cannot be, it is equally true that it has been demonstrated to be one of the most effective, at least, of all psychotherapies, discussed in Chapter 8. IPT has also been subjected to rigorous outcome research, but its application for chronic pain is wanting. We decided to show its relevance in treating a young person with chronic pain who had experienced serious health-related losses. The same can be said of family therapy, grief therapy, and others. They provide different levels of evidence, but judged against RCTs, they tend to fall short. Does that suggest that we await such evidence? We argue against such rigidity, and attempt to make a case in favor of treatment of choice determined by the weight of the problems presented by our patient. That is not to minimize the need for credible outcome research in any way.

We have one central reason for adopting the above proposition. To support our proposition, we can draw on our choice of task-centered therapy to treat a young man with chronic pain and multiple social and interpersonal problems. This particular therapy was developed to specifically address those issues. There is no question that task-centered approach is in urgent need of quantitative or qualitative support.

R. Roy, *Psychosocial Interventions for Chronic Pain*,
DOI:10.1007/978-0-387-76296-8_11 © Springer Science+Business Media, LLC 2008

We recognize the limitation, yet we argue that this therapy deserves our attention in dealing with some very specific problems and indeed credible outcome research.

We were impressed by the paucity of outcome research with many psychotherapies. We are inclined to make the following observation for this state of affairs. Psychotherapies that fall outside behavioral psychotherapies in general and CBT in particular fail to attract much research. It must be noted that the effectiveness of most of the therapies we have presented is backed by some research. SFT furnishes a good example. The therapy shows promise and the research methodology needs further refinement. Another point of note with SFT is its virtual absence of research with our population. The same observation can be made in relation to psychodynamic psychotherapy.

But, as noted, most nonbehavioral psychotherapies fall short of the APA-recommended definition of what may constitute acceptable methodology. The point needs to be made that RCTs and single-case designs with repeated multiple measures are expensive to implement. Should they be regarded as the last word in outcome research? Perhaps not. Qualitative methodology is increasingly assuming a higher level of sophistication. Controlled studies that fall short of RCTs should not be rejected out of hand. Even some uncontrolled studies deserve our attention.

It is noteworthy that psychotherapies have a history of being driven by guruism and the flavor of the day. We demonstrated this in our review of family therapy (Roy and Frankel, 1995). Psychoanalysis was certainly not research driven and at a personal level, when I trained in psychodynamic psychotherapy and systems-based family therapy, not one of my very learned supervisors ever raised the broader question of research evidence and effectiveness. "Faith of the counselor" in a particular therapeutic approach was and perhaps is the major determinant of the therapy we use in our practice. SFT gained enormous popularity before any evidence of its effectiveness, such as it is, emerged and, as we noted, this therapy awaits more and better quality outcome research. Nevertheless, the fact remains that, by and large, many of us tend to provide psychotherapy based on our training and bias rather than evidence of effectiveness.

In the final analysis research-driven psychotherapy has some way to go. A recent review of EBP by social workers in many Western countries produced a discouraging picture (Thyer and Kazi, 2004). There is only a vague awareness of the necessity of such practice and many faculties and schools of social work do not incorporate EBP in their graduate curriculum. Commenting on the future of EBP, Gambrill (2004) made the following observation: "Potential contribution of EBP (evidence-based practice) could be derailed by the justification approach to knowledge so common in the helping professions that encourages a search for data that support, validate and confirm what is believed. A robust literature shows that people tend to seek support for preferred views and ignore contradictory evidence and alternative views. Confirmatory biases contribute to inflated claims of what is known." In short, the wide adoption of EBP by the practitioners remains an uphill task. There also exists some political opposition to EBP as it is seen as a ploy by the government to ration therapy and contain cost. This may not be a tenable argument from the patient's point of view. Do we as therapists have an obligation to inform our patients about the effectiveness of treatment (therapy) before we ask them to invest time and sometimes money?

Our journey through the voluminous literature on psychotherapy failed to answer one critical question. How extensively is psychotherapy incorporated into the overall treatment for medically ill patients in general and chronic pain sufferers in particular? We are uncertain about the answer, but we are inclined to think that it is far from universal. The second issue that we alluded to in the preface about "one therapy (CBT) fits all" received considerable affirmation just based on the sheer volume of outcome research conducted to date on CBT. Although successful outcome of CBT with chronic pain sufferers is impressive, it is not a panacea.

Our third observation is the very limited research conducted to date with a whole range of psychotherapies with chronic pain sufferers. Family therapy, the use of which I have reported extensively, still awaits sound outcome research (Roy, 2006). IPT, the effectiveness of which has been demonstrated, is another case in point. In this context, even though SFT shows promise, its claims of success are perhaps somewhat inflated. More importantly, to date there is no research to test its effectiveness with chronic pain sufferers. SFT and task-centered therapy are specifically designed to directly address "social problems" and, as such, have much relevance in treating chronic pain patients. The field of psychotherapy remains wide open to methodologically sound research, innovation, and experimentation. It may be some time before EBP is the order of the day. However, one fact that is worthy of attention is our discovery of innovative treatment programs. One that stands out is a comprehensive pain management treatment plan that was created by bringing together all the key components in a community setting without the benefit of a centralized hospital-based program (Chapter 10). Innovation and research need to go hand in hand.

References

Fisher, J. and O'Donohue, W. (Eds.) (2006) Practitioner's Guide to Evidence-Based Psychotherapy. New York, Springer Science+Business Media, LLC.

Gambrill, E. (2004) The future of evidence-based social work practice. In: Thyer, B. and Kazi, M. (Eds.) International Perspective on Evidence-Based Practice in Social Work. Birmingham, UK, Venture Press.

McDaniel, S., Hepworth, J., and Doherty, W. (1992) Medical Family Therapy: A Biopsychosocial Approach to Family and Health Problems. New York, Basic Books.

Roy, R. (2006) Chronic Pain and Family: A Clinical Perspective. New York, Springer.

Roy, R. and Frankel, H. (1995) How Good is Family Therapy? Toronto, University of Toronto Press.

Thyer, B. and Kazi, M. (2004) International Perspective on Evidence-Based Practice in Social Work. Birmingham, UK, Venture Press.

Index

Printed in the United States of America